Never **Binge** Again™

Reprogram Yourself to Think Like a Permanently Thin Person™ on the Food Plan Of Your Choice!

DISCLAIMER: For education only. You are responsible for determining your own nutritional, medical, and psychological needs. If you require assistance with this task you must consult with a licensed physician, nutritionist, psychologist, and/ or other professional. No medical, psychological, and/or nutritional advice is offered through this book. Even though the author is a licensed psychologist, he does not offer psychological services, psychological advice and/or psychological counsel in his role as author of this book. In particular, if you have ever been diagnosed with an eating disorder you agree not to create your Food Plan and/ or any Food Rules without the input and approval of a psychiatrist, psychologist, and licensed dietician. Psy Tech Inc. and/or Never Ever Again, Inc. is only willing to license you the right to utilize this book in the event you agree with these terms. If you do not agree with these terms, please do not read the book, delete it from all electronic devices you own, and/or return it to your place of purchase for a full refund (where applicable).

ISBN: 151516294X and 13:9781515162940

CONTENTS

CHAPTER 1

The Outrageous Promise

"This can't possibly be true"
Sincerely, Your Fat-Thinking-Self

I'd like to make an outrageous, life-changing promise: Suspend judgment long enough to learn one *(somewhat crazy)* mental trick and you can achieve full control of your eating...*forever*.

NOT the painful, grit-your-teeth-and-bear-it control you've experienced while dieting before, but real control that lasts. Effortless control you feel secure about 24x7x365, without constant thought. Natural, lifelong control which represents true peace with food. So you can obtain the body you want, the health you deserve, and the sense of confidence and esteem which comes from sticking to a commitment.

Plus, once you learn this mental trick it will not only act to protect you against the thoughts which cause you to overeat today, but anything your "fat-thinking-self" might dream up tomorrow.

But fair warning: This trick-of-mind is fairly unusual, and you may have a negative reaction when you first hear it. Some people put the book down. Others call me a lunatic.

That's OK.

I don't mind the criticism because I know that my "strange" approach, although aggravating to some, has been extremely helpful to countless others...

Because what you've been calling a weight problem — *or difficulty sticking with your best thinking about what to eat* — is in reality a survival drive gone wrong. This is why all your rational attempts to keep to your commitments have failed, and why you keep getting derailed from your best-laid dietary and nutritional plans.

It's also why it seems like no matter how hard you try, you eventually find yourself eating in ways you swore you never would again. And it's why you may feel demoralized, dejected, and hopeless about ever successfully dealing with food.

When you start to rein in this survival-drive-run-amuck, it's going to fear for its life. But thankfully, there's ONE insight to which this seemingly unconquerable drive responds. One which can help you utterly dominate it, giving you full control of your eating from now on.

So feel free to entertain every critical voice in your head. In fact, becoming aware of your internal objections is an essential part of the process. I've actually set up the book to stimulate them.

All I'm asking is you give this a chance.

Give it a full read and promise yourself to withhold judgment. Try it out for a while, even if it seems nutty or doesn't quite work for you at first. If at that point you still think this idea is just not for you, that's fine. By then, you'll have made a fully informed decision, which is critical because — *as you'll soon realize* — this is about a lot more than losing a few pounds. And it's about more than your health.

This is about accomplishing all your goals and dreams with more confidence and security than you ever thought possible.

What's at stake is everything you care about, as it is for everyone who's ever really struggled with food. And if you'll just pause to breathe for a moment, I know you'll nod your head in agreement. At minimum, you'll have to acknowledge how important it is to get control of this eating thing once and for all.

So please keep your mind as open as it's ever been.

After all... *what if I'm right?*

WHO AM I?

I'm a formerly obese guy with very poor cardiovascular genetics...

A guy who almost ate himself to death despite a dozen warnings from doctors and other health professionals...

Who wasted years of his life believing he had a mysterious disease which caused him to compulsively overeat...

And who used to think he was powerless to resist bagels, pizza, chocolate, donuts, pasta, potato chips, and pretty much anything else which tasted good in mass quantities.

My ongoing food compulsions and preoccupations did not deter me, however, from earning a Ph.D. in clinical psychology, nor from building a large, very successful practice, nor even from funding my own food-preference research project with 40,000+ people.

And for over 25 years I was the CEO of companies which provided tens of millions of dollars in research and consulting services to Fortune 500 firms including major food manufacturers like Lipton, Kraft, Nabisco, etc.

Frankly, I'm a guy who couldn't stop thinking about food, even while he was working with psychotherapy patients and coaching clients...

Someone who spent most of his life feeling desperate to control his food problem. That is, until I discovered a child-like trick of mind which got me thinking like a permanently thin person...

A weird idea which got in my head and grew progressively stronger by itself, no matter how hard my fat-thinking-self tried to eliminate it!

WARNING:
Your Fat Thinking Alter-Ego Does
NOT Want You to Read This Book!

Your Fat-Thinking-Self will say anything to prevent you from reading this. For example, it may already be saying something like this:

> "You've got to be kidding me! Another diet plan? There's NO way we could ever do this. You're too weak, you never stick with a hard and fast food rule. Besides, are we really just going to eat like rabbits for the rest of our life? C'mon. Just put the book down and let's go have us a little Bingeing party. Can we? Can we? Huh!!?"

So let me promise you something up front: This book is about cementing your ability to stick with the Food Plan of your choice. It's not about getting you to follow *(or not follow)* any particular diet. Absolutely everything about what you eat, when you eat, and where you eat will be entirely up to you.

Your Fat-Thinking-Self will also object to drawing the clear "lines in the sand" required by this technique:

> "Are you really NEVER going to cross the line again? That's just a set up for feeling guilty when you Binge and you know it. Do you really need more guilt in your life? Now just go get me some 'comfort food'...it'll be yummy!" – Your Fat Thinking Self

These guilt-threats need not frighten or control you. Because in this book we'll apply a very kindhearted, effective way to recover from mistakes without becoming preoccupied with guilt and shame. If you fall down, you'll just get up and resume where you left off. There's NO need to repeatedly smack yourself in the head with a spatula! *(Note your Fat-Thinking-Self's immediate excitement at the possibility of you falling down.)*

That said, since fear of guilt and failure stops many people before they've had a chance to really try this, let's talk a bit about how we'll handle mistakes in the Never Binge Again way of thinking. In short, we just treat ourselves the same way we'd treat a child who's genuinely trying to accomplish something important.

For example, suppose your 5 year old daughter has her heart set on riding her bicycle to the top of a very steep hill without stopping. Would you say "You'll never get to the top without stopping, little Sarah. That hill is WAY too steep. I don't want you to feel guilty and ashamed after you fail, so let's not even try, OK?"

Of course not! Instead, you'd help her set her sights on the goal with confidence and enthusiasm. And if she didn't make it, you'd be right by her side to figure out what went wrong so she could do better next time. You certainly wouldn't make her feel guilty for failing to reach the top, nor prevent her from setting the goal in the first place.

In this scenario, Sarah would know in her heart of hearts that if she did fail, you'd be right there to pick up the pieces and help her do better next time. But—*and this is the key*—with your support and enthusiasm she'd pedal up the hill with confidence and determination. And eventually—*perhaps not on the first few tries*—she WOULD make it...in large part because you protected her from becoming pre-occupied with the possibility of failure.

In a way, you'd have encouraged Sarah to purposefully "keep a secret" from herself, so that doubt and insecurity would not interfere with her energy and concentration on the goal.

In my experience this is the mindset of people who stop bingeing. Like little Sarah confidently pedaling up that big hill, you'll learn to put even the remotest possibility of failure out of your mind...even if you DO at times fail on any given attempt. If you make a mistake, you'll just pick yourself up and get back to pedaling in the right direction, speaking kindly to yourself the whole time.

It's almost impossible to Binge if you refuse to yell at yourself. And if you DO resolve to get up if you happen to fail, no matter how many times, you can't help but eventually get to the top.

Uncertainty, doubt, and low self-esteem are the psychological cancers which fuel overeating behavior. But rather than take years to eliminate these problems using traditional psychological methods, we're going to cut right to the chase, remove the possibility of failure from our minds as we "pedal up that hill," and quickly face down the guilt if we happen to make a mistake.

Therefore, we can confidently tell your Fat Thinking Self it no longer has the power to undermine your efforts with the fear of failure, guilt, and shame. With the power of Never Binge Again you can set any reasonable food goal with confidence and keep pursuing it until you achieve it—no matter how many attempts it may require. (At this point your Fat Thinking Self will get very excited about the possibility of you requiring multiple attempts to stop bingeing. Just ignore these thoughts for now)

We'll go into more detail about dealing with the fear of failure, guilt about mistakes, etc. later in the book, but now that you understand the basic concept it should be a lot easier for you to keep reading.

There's one last objection your Fat-Thinking-Self will raise about this book to stop you from finishing it, however: It will suggest aggressively rejecting all your fat-thoughts is a form of self-cruelty. It would prefer you keep trying to "love yourself thin" instead.

I promise you'll be loving yourself MORE—and beating yourself up LESS—when we're done.

In this context, it's very important you understand that...

It's Almost Impossible to "Love Yourself Thin!"

Identifying and caging your fat-thinking alter-ego is how YOU finally come to dominate all your food decisions and permanently reprogram yourself to think like a thin person. It's how to disempower the destructive thinking which has, to this point, caused you so much trouble with food.

As noted above, many people reject this mental maneuver because they want to love ALL parts of themselves, no matter what.

The problem with loving, feeding, and nurturing ALL your thoughts and feelings is certain impulses are too strong to restrain when they're given even a tiny opening. For many people, the physical and biochemical set up when it comes to food and other survival drives makes it extremely difficult to "love themselves thin." In my experience this includes *most* people who struggle with binge-eating and/or serious bouts of overeating.

The compassionate soul inside me wishes this weren't true...

But our "overeating and binging" thoughts are indeed a part of us. So I understand why people may perceive this technique as unnecessarily harsh at first. But if you'll take the time to think about it, I know you'll agree these thoughts represent the most reckless, most juvenile part of us...

The part which has repeatedly caused us to act against our own best judgment, and continually change our minds about our most serious food commitments.

These thoughts are worthy of permanent rejection.

In my experience, the act of recovering from Bingeing, serious overeating, and/or simply learning to stick to a diet is NOT like nurturing a wounded animal back to health. It's more like capturing and caging an aggressive Doberman Pincher. This dog must respect and obey you—or it will have its way every time!

Interrupting and disempowering the thoughts which sustain your bingeing and overeating is not a game of mercy, it's a game of unbreakable control and domination.

The fundamental reason people keep changing their minds about food commitments is because they are unknowingly giving their "fat-thinking-self" nurturance and love.

For all the reasons above, the mental entity which will hereafter house ALL your fat thinking shall be deemed "the Pig!™"

WHAT IS 'THE PIG'?

THE FIRST THING YOU NEED TO KNOW IS THIS: THE PIG IS NOT YOU!

Your Pig™ is NOT you!

The second thing you need to know is you can call it by a different name like "junkyard dog", "feral cat", "inner food demon"... or anything else which doesn't remind you of a cute pet... because you're going to want to distance yourself from it, NOT love and nurture it...

But I call my fat thinking self 'The Pig', so for the sake of the discussion here, I'll address the seemingly uncontrollable urge to eat as 'The Pig'.

Here's what separates YOU from 'The Pig'...

You have dreams and aspirations, but the Pig lives only to Binge.

You enjoy everything life has to offer, but the Pig wants only its junk and will say whatever it takes to get you to feed it...

The Pig doesn't care about the consequences to your health, body, well-being, or happiness — because the Pig must get its stuff at any cost! You want to love, learn, laugh, and live your life to the fullest. But the Pig lives only for that "one more" precious Binge.

You can plan, organize, and accomplish amazing things. But the Pig sees life as one big food party and spends all its time and energy trying to convince you to indulge.

Thankfully, YOU are the only one who can feed it.

Understand this and you're half way to controlling your weight forever.

The other half is learning to *cold-heartedly* ignore its Squeals.

When it comes down to it, either you or the Pig is going to suffer, and it's NOT going to be you!

Your Inner Pig™ is responsible for a LOT of the misery in your life...

It convinced you to eat all the wrong foods, in the wrong portions, at the wrong times — downgrading your health, confidence, and quality of life most likely for decades by the time you became willing to read this.

The Pig has talked you out of every perfectly reasonable weight-loss plan you've ever made...

It's prevented you from nourishing your body, mind, and soul...

It's robbed you of not only the body you want, but the energy you need to build the life of your dreams.

It's the Pig that's caused you to live with this unnecessary weight burden...

It's the Pig that's drained your success, health, and happiness...

And it's the Pig that's making you feel hopeless about ever losing weight for good.

But the Pig couldn't care less.

It cares ONLY for its own pleasure, and will destroy everything you love without blinking an eye... just to get one more precious bite.

The Pig deserves NO love and NO compassion.

It is NOT your inner child, a cute little pet, or anything else YOU might truly value in life.

So don't you dare confuse "pig" *(small 'p')* with the Pig *(capital 'P!')*...

Because pigs *(the real animals)* are quite loving and adorable. Some people even keep them as pets. And in the REAL world, they need our help and protection...

But the "Pig" *(with a capital 'P')* is an out-of-control eating machine which will destroy everything you love if you let it.

Unfortunately, we can't completely eliminate it from our lives because the Pig is intimately connected to an anatomical structure we need to survive *(the midbrain)*. But you can eternally dominate it as long as you don't confuse its Squeals for your own desires, and as long as you do what's otherwise necessary for your survival.

THE PIG IS NOT YOU!

As crazy as it sounds, you must learn to treat the Pig with the same distaste and disrespect you'd feel for a BULLY. Because every time you "cross the line" and Binge despite your best-laid plans, there's actually a little voice inside you — *the Pig's voice* — working hard to make it "OK". And the Pig (the Bully) doesn't care how sick it makes you, how much pain it causes, and/or how much it derails your best laid plans to achieve important goals.

All the Pig cares about is convincing you it's perfectly OK to eat a whole LOT of garbage...

But it's NOT OK! And this trick of mind is how you finally get fed up with the internal thoughts which—*until now*— have been ruining so much of your life in exchange for a few moments of toxic pleasure.

For this reason, we're going to voluntarily and aggressively separate ourselves from the Pig in our own mental space, and in so doing we're going to gain 100% dominance over its destructive ideas.

The Pig is NOT you, and deserves NO respect. Learn to hear its Squeals, then promptly ignore them.

AM I A RAVING LUNATIC?

Not quite.

I don't believe there's a REAL pig inside anyone.

It's only a mental concept. A voluntary trick of mind.

But here's the thing: It's not "just" a trick of mind, it's THE trick of mind that works where others fail!

We may wish to acknowledge the trick in order to maintain our ability to think rationally. But in order to get the job done, once we've acknowledged this, it becomes imperative to treat the Pig as if it were real.

Therefore, this will be the only time I'll point out the Pig doesn't really exist.

It's a conceptual framework to help you separate from the thoughts and feelings which, until now, have derailed your best-laid plans. A way of thinking which helps you take control and live the life you deserve. But in order for it to work, it's got to seem 100% real to us during ALL potential moments of temptation.

You might struggle with this idea at first. Your Pig would certainly prefer you believed it didn't exist. Because then you'd think its Squeals were your own thoughts — and, as you'll soon discover, this is the ONLY way the Pig can get you to feed it.

Who cares...

Cage the Pig and tell it to shut up!

REMEMBER: It's your mind and you're allowed to organize your thoughts and feelings any way you want. The Pig exists because you SAY it exists, end of story.

"Are you really taking any of this nonsense seriously? C'mon... let's just go Binge!"
Sincerely - Your Pig

TAKE THE TEST:
Is It Worth Defining a "Fat Thinking Alter-Ego" Inside You?

If you're not sure whether you're ready to define a "Fat Thinking Alter Ego" *(Pig)* from which to aggressively separate, find out how much damage it's already done by taking the test at www. NeverBingeAgain.com *(Available after you sign up for the FREE reader bonuses)*

ALTERNATIVE NAMES FOR YOUR PIG

Even though I carefully explain "The Pig" is really just a moniker for your Lizard brain and is NOT you any more so than your ovaries *(or testes)*...

Some people hate naming a part of themselves – The 'Pig' because it brings back painful memories and feels like self-abuse...

If that's the case with you, you should avoid naming your fat thinking self the 'Pig'. As mentioned previously, there are plenty of other names you can use, like junkyard dog, feral cat, the saboteur and others. Some of my clients like to call their enemy an "Inner Slacker™" which "Whispers™ for its Junk™"

If you DO choose to use an alternate name, however, it WILL slightly alter the terms you'll want to use for the rest of the system. For example, you'll soon learn to refer to those things your Inner Pig wants you to eat as "Pig Slop™"... but if you're referring to YOUR inner enemy as a junkyard dog you can instead call these things "Trash"...

Also, you'll soon see we call the irrational voice your Pig uses to convince you to eat Pig Slop "Pig Squeal™"... but, following the same metaphor, you can just refer to it as Whining or Groveling...

See where I'm going?

Just don't choose a cutesy name for your out-of-control-fat-thinking-self.

The name must accurately represent an aggressive, manipulative bully which cares only about making you eat badly and nothing else...

So you'll be able to discipline and control this part of yourself without feeling remorse and/or unease.

Finally... I will continue to use term 'the Pig' throughout this book, simply because it's the name I've personally picked for my own Lizard Brain run amuck with food.

WHY WE MUST DISCIPLINE AND CONTROL VS. LOVE OUR INNER FOOD DEMON

It's important you know I'm a compassionate guy, and I DO believe in nurturing our inner wounded child... just NOT for the purpose of overcoming overeating.

I WANT you to feel loved.

I WANT you to self-actualize.

I WANT you to love yourself more...

And if you need a hug, well... I'm just a big teddy bear and I'll be the first guy to give it to you...

But 30+ years of painful experience trying the "love yourself thin" approach—*including a self-funded study with thousands of participants AND working directly with hundreds of clients*—has convinced me beyond a shadow of a doubt that this is NOT the way to arrest serious overeating and binging difficulties.

There are four reasons. The first is our neuroanatomy.

See, our brains evolved in three distinct parts *(And yes, I'm dramatically oversimplifying for illustration)*...

> **The Lizard Brain** *(Brain Stem)* is the oldest part. When it sees something in the environment it says to itself "Do I eat it, do I mate with it, or do I kill it!?" There's NO interest in family, love, or relationships. No accounting for long term goals, spirituality, art, or music. It's just "eat, mate, or kill." This is the part which takes over when your diet flies out the window for a momentary indulgence. The Lizard Brain, when misdirected towards bad foods, IS your Pig.

> **The Mammalian Brain** evolved after the lizard brain to ensure the wellbeing of the family. Essentially it's job is to say to the Lizard Brain: "Wait! Don't eat, mate, or kill that thing until we know it's good for the tribe too!" This is the seat of emotion which bonds and binds you to others in the world.

> **And the Neocortex or "Logical Brain"** came last to control the Lizard and Mamallian Brain in favor of longer term goals... things like weight loss and fitness... but also the human notions of love, self-identify, spirituality, music, art, etc.

The Mammalian brain can inhibit the Lizard Brain...

And the Logical Brain *(Neocortex)* can inhibit both the Lizard and the Mammalian Brain...

This is evolution's design, which allows us to regulate ANY impulse. We are NOT powerless! But when you try to "love yourself thin", "nurture your inner wounded child", and/or "figure out what's eating you" the moment you experience a craving, what you're actually doing is relinquishing tens of millions of years of control evolution has provided your Neocortex with and just allowing the Lizard brain to take over.

Loving the Lizard brain *(your Inner Pig)* at the moment of impulse MINIMIZES your ability to control it!

Instead, cultivate a sense of distaste for it so you can get those extra microseconds you need to wake up and make the right decisions.

But beyond our neuroanatomy, we are all facing an overwhelming, perfect storm of socio-economic forces from which we need to set ourselves squarely apart. What's required is for us to become fed up and angry, NOT lovingly complacent.

To place this in context I'd like to briefly review a set of very powerful studies done by scientific experimenters Peter Milner and James Olds in the late 1950s. Although these experiments would clearly not be ethical from an animal rights perspective today *(or perhaps even when they WERE done)*, they do nevertheless illustrate a critical point: Mammals will engage in severe self-neglect in order to obtain artificial stimulation of their neurological pleasure centers.

Here's what was done...

The experimenters implanted electrodes in the pleasure centers of the brain in a group of rats... then connected those electrodes to a button the rats could press to activate it.

The results were dramatic. The rats would press the button thousands of times per hour to self-stimulate. They preferred self-stimulation to food and water *(even when they were hungry and thirsty)*...

Male rats would ignore a female in heat in order to keep self-stimulating. They would also cross shock-grids on the floor, enduring significant pain, to get to their lever.

Female rats would abandon their nursing pups in order to press the lever.

Some rats did nothing but press the lever thousands of times per hour for an entire day. And the researchers had to forcefully unhook these rats from the apparatus in order to stop them from starving themselves!

Studies in humans have borne out similar results. *(Moan and Heath)*

What these studies tell us is it's entirely possible to use artificial means to hijack our survival drive against our best interests.

Which brings me to reason #2 we need to tackle our food problems with a much more aggressive approach...

In my not-so-humble opinion Big Food uses artificial means to hijack OUR survival drives for profit. The rats felt they couldn't live without their pleasure buttons and willingly neglected their nutritional needs *(and everything else which is traditionally important to a rat)* to keep pressing them. Similarly, people in our society feel they can't live without the "pleasure buttons" provided by industrial food's bags, boxes, and containers... and will fight to keep pressing these buttons at the dire expense of their health needs.

The economic force of Big Food has trumped nutrition and hijacked our survival drive.

Then, of course, Big Advertising spends billions to convince us these food-like-substances are irresistible *(and even good for us)*. Did you know there are 5,000+ food messages beamed at us via TV, Radio, and the internet every year but hardly ANY of them are for fruit and vegetables?...

Oh, and lest you think you're immune because advertising "doesn't work on" you, here's a very disturbing fact: Advertising works BETTER on people who think they're immune because their sales resistance is down! *(It's a little evil when you stop to think about it)*

That's force #3... Big Advertising.

Then, the Addiction Treatment Industry *(force #4)* tells us we're "powerless" over our addictions, we've got a chronic, progressive, mysterious disease against which there is often no human defense, and the best we can every hope for is to abstain one day at a time. This message is readily absorbed by our culture to the point many of us believe we CAN'T give up our pleasure buttons even if we want to!

Summarizing...

Big Food puts as much starch, sugar, oil, sodium, fat, excitotoxins, and other chemical stimulants into a small space as they legally can...

Then they package it up to APPEAR healthy and irresistible...

Big Advertising makes us believe it...

Big Addiction Treatment says we're powerless to resist...

And we walk around thinking we're just supposed to love ourselves more when the urge hits!

Is it any wonder we've got a worldwide obesity epidemic on our hands?

But there's very good news...

You CAN set yourself apart from all this with a simple set of techniques. You only need to learn to recognize your Inner Pig's voice when it Squeals *(or your Inner Junkyard Dog's voice when it Whines and Whimpers, etc.)*... and then summarily ignore it, while ensuring you're getting more than enough healthy nutrition elsewhere.

FAIR WARNING BEFORE YOU READ ANY FURTHER:

I AM GOING TO TALK ABOUT YOUR "INNER PIG" THROUGHOUT THIS WHOLE BOOK: How to capture and cage and dominate it. It's my strong experience that people develop MORE self-esteem and self-love when they find themselves finally able to control their eating behavior and accomplish their goals. The Pig metaphor is the best one I've found for at least half the people with whom I've worked.

However...

IF ALL MY "INNER PIG" TALK IS GOING TO BOTHER YOU, PLEASE STOP READING RIGHT NOW! OTHERWISE YOU'RE ONLY GOING TO BECOME ANGRY AND GIVE ME BAD REVIEWS, ETC.

But if you're intrigued and open minded...

And you CAN see the value in aggressively separating your human self from your lizard brain in your own mind...

And if the Pig metaphor DOES bother you, you promise to just adjust the language and call it something else...

Then please read on, because this very well could be the thing that works for you after all these years of struggling!

(If you're still reading I'll assume we do NOT have a problem so this is the last time I'll "apologize" for using Pig language, OK?)

How to hear the Pig's Squeals

To truly dominate the Pig we need to distinguish its Squeals from our own rational hunger. You'll need to make a concrete Food Plan with your own specific Food Rules *(even JUST ONE rule to get started)... and then definitively commit.*

The Pig hates rules and will do its very best to destroy the integrity of any you may set. This is why you must take 100% ownership and responsibility. It's also why every rule—*and your Food Plan as a whole*—must be set with 100% clarity. Otherwise, the Pig can use "fuzzy lines" and "diets you're just trying out for a while" to mercilessly assail your integrity and confidence.

You simply must...

Create your own Food Plan

You'll need to thoroughly embrace your own Food Plan, comprised solely of your own Food Rules. Why yours and not some diet guru's, nutritionist's, and/or weight loss doctor's? Because after you're five years old nobody can follow you around making sure you eat right, that's why.

Of course, you can and should get expert advice.

By all means, read health books, and work with experts you trust to inform your thinking. But if you're reading *this* book, odds are you've already done so. In fact, I'd be willing to bet my left kidney—*and I'm rather fond of that one*—you've got a pretty good idea of what a well-balanced, nourishing, and reasonable diet looks like.

It'd work too, if you'd only stick to it!

So let's skip all the "Mama said eat your vegetables" stuff and cut right to the "stick to it" part...

If you're finally going to stick to a plan, you'll need to OWN it — 100%.

After all, whose hands are going to grab the car keys, start the engine, drive to the market, put the food in the cart, take out the money, give it to the cashier, put the bags in the trunk, bring them inside, put them away, choose the meals, prepare them, get out the fork, stick it in, pick it up to your lips and put it in your mouth?

Yours.

Not your doctor's, nutritionist's, diet guru's, or therapist's hands, that's for sure! And it's a good thing, too, because for all their well-meaning advice and expertise, none of these people could follow you around 24 hours a day, even if they wanted to do so.

The ONLY way you're ever going to succeed is if you accept 100% responsibility for every bite and swallow. You see, "trying out" professional diet plans is a type of dependency which sets the Pig up to retake control like this:

> "Must've been a bad diet plan that nutritionist, doctor, or diet-guru recommended. You'll have to talk to them about it. Or maybe we need to find someone else to follow. Oh well, in the meantime we might as well just Binge. Yummy!!!" — Sincerely, Your Pig

So, this one's up to you. You're completely and utterly responsible — 100%, not 99.999%. ONE HUNDRED PERCENT. Get it?

Breathe for a moment here and listen for your Pig's inevitable Squeal:

> "Wait just a minute here! This book itself is a diet book too, isn't it? After all Glenn's just another guy trying to make a buck with weight-loss advice. So go ahead, try it out for a while. Sooner or later you'll cheat like you always do, and then I'll be free to Binge again. Why wait? Let's do it NOW! Yippee!!!" – Sincerely, Your Pig

What a Pig. Cage the Pig!

How to own your Food Plan 100%

This might seem obvious but...

The best way to own your Food Plan is to write it down.

Every single Food rule... and the Plan as a whole.

100%, unambiguously.

That means, if 10 people were to review your plan and watch how you ate all day long, they'd *unanimously* agree whether you were on it or off it. Not 9 of them. ALL of them.

However, your Food Plan is a very private matter. So this "would 10 people agree" test is only a thought experiment to help YOU judge whether you've articulated it clearly and precisely.

The reason you want to spell out your plan with enough precision that 10 people could agree is because ambiguity is the Pig's best friend...

Ambiguity is a yellow light, not a red one...

And the Pig will go 100 miles per hour from a quarter mile away to speed through a yellow light. You can count on it, every time.

When the specifics are laid out in incontrovertible detail, however, you convert fuzzy yellow lights into red, and it becomes impossible for the Pig to run the light without getting caught—because you'll immediately recognize any thought suggesting you run the light as Pig Squeal *(fat thinking)*...

...which you can promptly ignore — not argue or debate with, not console, not attend to in any way...

Ignore.

There's NO use trying to reason with The Pig. It doesn't care for your well-being. All it wants is to Binge, and it will twist around every last bit of information and attention you provide in order to persuade you to feed it. Therefore, we starve the Pig of information and attention at every turn.

If you simply ignore the Pig, the red lights will hold forever.

Why?

Because YOU are the only one who can put your foot on the gas and run the lights — *no matter how much the Pig may protest or try to convince you otherwise.*

The only danger is in not recognizing Pig's Squeal for what it is. *The only danger is thinking the Pig is you.* That's why we're such sticklers for a precisely defined plan.

You do NOT have to follow anyone else's guidelines for writing up your Food Plan. Do it in whatever manner suits you best.

After all, it's your Plan. And as long as it's 100% unambiguous, clear, and nutritionally sound, it will suffice.

In a moment, I'll provide a simple set of guidelines for constructing your Food Plan. However, I must first warn you, your Pig will Squeal louder in response to this part of the book than any other. Just continue to ignore its objections and remember four important things:

> ➤ (1) Even though we'll be talking about how to use "Never" and "Always" kinds of rules to provide clarity, these are NOT required elements of this program—*you can construct healthy and effective Food Plans entirely without them. (Download the free food plan starter templates from* www.NeverBingeAgain.com *for examples)...*

> ➤ (2) The goal is to create the *LEAST* severe Food Plan which still protects you from previously troublesome food behaviors. Only you can know how to comprise this. But the purpose of the plan is to give you an unshakable sense of confidence, not turn you into a "Food Nazi"...

> ➤ (3) Even though we'll push any semblance of a doubt in our ability to keep to your Food Plan out of our minds so we can "pedal up the hill" with 100% confidence, we do have a plan for gently forgiving ourselves and quickly resuming course if mistakes are made.

> ➤ (4) You don't have to create the whole Food Plan at once. In fact, most people do better by creating just ONE Food Rule to address their single most troublesome trigger food and/or food behavior... with NO concern about losing weight. Only then—*after playing the Never Binge Again™ game successfully for a few weeks to a few months and reclaiming their sense of hope, enthusiasm, and power!*—do they venture forth into a full Food Plan with a multitude of

rules. *(And, generally speaking, only then do they also begin to adjust these rules to include weight loss as a goal. Stop binging and gaining weight first. Get control. Reclaim your power. Lose weight later.)*

With this framework in mind, let's talk about:

A Simple Set of Guidelines for Constructing a Food Plan

As long as your Food Plan is easy to remember, unambiguous, and nutritionally complete you *can* make it work. Here are some simple categories of Food Rules you may wish to consider:

> **NEVERS:** What foods, drinks, and behaviors will you *never* indulge in again as long as you live?

> **ALWAYS:** What will you *always* do regarding food, drink, and food behaviors? *(For example "I always eat six servings of fruit and vegetables each calendar day" or "I always write down what I may potentially eat the next day before I go to bed to force myself to think through any difficult spots.")*

> **UNRESTRICTED:** What foods, drinks, and food behaviors will you permit yourself to have *without restriction?*

> **CONDITIONALS:** What foods, drinks, and behaviors will you permit only at certain times, in certain amounts, and/ or restricted by other *conditions? (Specify these in exquisite detail so there's no ambiguity about when the light is red vs. green. Avoid yellow lights because in the Pig's way of thinking, yellow = bright green.)*

There are a lot of different variables involved in constructing a Food Plan, so it's somewhat more difficult to quit Bingeing than to stop abusing drugs, cigarettes, or alcohol. With the latter you can just quit. But with food, you've got to keep eating *something*.

The Pig will try to defeat you with this fact. A good Food Plan eliminates the possibility.

Once you're armed with a crystal clear plan, you'll quickly catch on to your Pig's handful of sneaky strategies, no matter how long you've previously been fooled. Therefore, we're going to spend considerable time illustrating how to adopt Nevers, Always, Unrestricteds, and Conditionals, and make them stick.

Let's start with NEVER.

Never is the simplest and clearest red light of all. Creating even one Never is a great way to learn how to hear the Pig's Squeals because it clearly draws the line between your food vs. Pig Slop. Setting even one Never is how you begin your new life.

> "OK, OK. If you're going to insist on doing something to slow down for a while, how about we just quit Bingeing one day at a time? I could definitely live with *that*. But whatever you do just don't say NEVER!"
> - Sincerely, Your Pig

How to Never Do Something (Anything) Again

NEVER is a word you won't hear much in our culture when it comes to food, alcohol, drugs, or any other pleasurable substance. That's a shame, because it's one of the most powerful words for taking permanent control over the Pig.

If you can't say you'll NEVER do *something* again *(or never engage in a particular food behavior again)*, the Pig knows it's only a matter of time until it gains the upper hand. If we define a "Binge" as engaging in any eating behavior which contradicts your Food Plan, then at very minimum we must be able to say we will NEVER Binge again.

So we will carefully define a livable and acceptable Food Plan and then NEVER break it again!

If you think about it, it's very odd how unwilling we've become to say NEVER when it comes to things which have caused so much misery in our lives. There are many behaviors we expect people never to engage in. So why not add one more when you have so much to gain?

> We expect responsible members of society to NEVER kill, rape, or steal...

> We expect people with life threatening allergies to avoid certain substances for the rest of their lives *(for example, there are some people who simply can't eat peanuts... EVER)*...

> We expect people to NEVER act on their sexual impulses in public...

> And married persons are supposed to confine their romantic and sexual adventures to each other. We even have a legal contract — *the marriage license* — which formalizes this understanding.

In fact, we've all learned to NEVER do many things just to get through everyday life:

> Never put your hand on a hot stove or in the electric socket

> Never threaten a political official with bodily harm

> Never grab a knife on the sharp end

And some of our 'Nevers' are so strongly ingrained we don't even realize they're learned behaviors. For example:

> Never pass gas at the table when dining with others

> Never grab a total stranger and kiss them on the lips

> Never sit at the teacher's desk in school

➢ Never take off your shoes and socks in church

➢ Never kick a policeman in the tushy

By the time most children are 10 years old they've naturally learned all of these things — and if they can do it, so can you. Adding one more 'Never' is child's play, no matter how much short-term pleasure one must sacrifice, and no matter what your Pig says!

"Are you really going to let this guy tell us to NEVER eat something again? C'mon, have a spine!!" – Sincerely, Your Fat Thinking Pig

IMPORTANT: Despite what your Pig may say, nobody is telling you what to do. In fact, that's the whole point.

Until now you've allowed the Pig to impose its will as if you were its slave. The information in this section gives YOU the power to make *permanent* decisions without the Pig's pernicious influence. The moment you put even one Never in your Food Rules, you've begun to cage the Pig!

Always

Always is Never's best friend. Defining some things you will ALWAYS do — *and acting on these commitments* — will give you even more confidence in your ability to cage the Pig.

Yes ALWAYS — you know, as in every day for the rest of your life.

Your 'Always' list can include general self-care in addition to food specific behaviors. For example, maybe you always start the day with a glass of water. Or maybe you always shower in the evening to help you get to sleep without extra food. Maybe you always meditate, exercise, or make fresh vegetable juice.

Maybe you always eat an apple before lunch...

Or maybe you don't *always* do anything.

Whatever you put here, just remember "always" and "never" are sacred vows. They become something the Pig can't assail, no matter how hard it tries, because the motives behind any Squeal suggesting an exception will be recognized immediately.

But as soon as you declare an intention which interferes with the Pig's yummy Binges, it will begin trying hard to defeat you. That's its job. You see, the Pig genuinely believes it will die without its precious stuff. But you will prevail as long as you remember the Pig Squeals are not your own thinking.

For example, suppose you always drink 16 ounces of purified water when you wake up in the morning. Always! As soon as you declare this rule, your Pig may say something like:

> "You can't say ALWAYS! How could you ever know that? One morning you'll wake up and forget. Or maybe you just won't feel like it. Some mornings you simply won't have the time. Then you'll have broken your silly vow. These ridiculous rules obviously don't matter since you can't possibly stick with them. We might as well just go BINGE!" —Sincerely, Your Pig

To prevail, you need only dismiss this as Pig Squeal.

Don't argue with the Pig.

Don't try to win a rational debate.

You don't need to, because the Pig is powerless to do anything without your consent. If the Pig could act on its own behalf it would immediately do so without asking. The very fact it talks *at all* proves its only hope is to convince you with its lies.

All that's necessary is to ignore it.

Notwithstanding this, let's dispute its points one by one, just to show you how ridiculous the Pig's arguments can be:

"You can't possibly mean 'Always'. Nobody can ever know what they're always going to do!"

This is the Pig's first attempt to pull the wool over your eyes. It says "You can't always do *anything!*" What a negative, confidence-destroying message.

Would you ever tell a young child: "Listen little Bobby, there's NO hope of remembering to brush your teeth, tie your shoes, and get dressed all by yourself every day. Just get that idea out of your head. You might as well just give up and accept you'll be a dependent little child the rest of your life... no matter what the big boys do."

Of course you wouldn't! Then why let the Pig talk to you that way?

The truth is there are many, many things people ALWAYS do daily...

> ➢ They turn off their alarm

> ➢ Roll out of bed

> ➢ Pee in the toilet

> ➢ Brush their teeth

> ➢ Etc.

> ➢ You can add one more ALWAYS anytime you want!

Let's go on...

"One morning you'll wake up and forget. And then you'll have broken your silly vow."

The Pig wants you to *plan to forget* your vow. But the very nature of a vow is a *plan to remember*. Which is more constructive? Which is more likely to improve your life?

The answer is obvious. So why would anyone ever make a plan to forget when we, as human beings, have the ability to plan to remember? People don't do that. Pigs do!

Any doubt you have about your ability to ALWAYS do something is 100% driven by the Pig's desire to have you break your vow. It doesn't care what impact this has on your confidence, self-esteem, health, or loved ones. The Pig is an anarchist and will try to destroy any structure which interferes with its Binges — at the expense of all your goals and aspirations. It has only contempt for your higher plans. Which is why we owe it nothing but contempt in return.

The truth is there are many things we're perfectly capable of remembering to do every single day. For example, taking care of our children.

> "Sorry little Sarah, I'm afraid I won't be giving you anything to eat or drink today. And you'll just have to stay up all night because Daddy can't possibly remember to put you to bed either" — *How your Pig would take care of a small child*

We also drive our cars home every day and park them in a safe spot – *instead of the lawn or the neighbor's rose garden* – even though the latter might be more convenient. We eat and/or drink enough to sustain us through one more day. And we put ourselves to bed every night somewhere at least reasonably safe and comfortable *(as opposed to lying down outside in our front yards without a tent or sleeping bag)*

> "These rules are just silly... obviously they don't matter at all since you can't possibly stick with them."

See how the Pig attempts to undermine even your simplest effort at positive, healthy change? It doesn't care if you die of dehydration. It must subvert your confidence and impulse control or else it won't get any more Pig Slop *(ever)*. Knowing this, it's clear we can't ever take it seriously.

> "You might as well just let me BINGE!"

The Pig's true nature comes out at last. The Binge is all it was after all along.

But just for argument's sake, suppose you DID break your plan to always drink 16 ounces of purified water every morning. Does it naturally follow you should go out and buy several bags of Doritos, a box of donuts, a pound of chocolate bars... and go to town on them all at once?

Of course not. If you forget to brush your teeth one morning, are you obligated to pick up a hammer and bang them all out? It's ridiculous.

Pig Squeal may *seem* rational on its surface, but it never is. (Never —as in never, ever, ever, ever, ever, EVER!)

The Pig can appear very appealing *at first* because of its ability to leverage a vulnerability in your survival drive. But when you hold its Squeal up to the light of day it NEVER makes any sense.

Just ignore Pig Squeal when you hear it. Period, end of story.

Unrestricted

Some people find it helpful to list out those things they can eat and/or drink in unlimited quantities without concern. Others just designate the 'Unrestricted' category as being everything that is not specifically listed on their restricted list.

Usually the 'Unrestricted' category is comprised of healthy "go to" foods you feel good about eating. For example, perhaps you want to allow as many leafy greens, cruciferous vegetables, green tea, beans, berries, clean water, etc., as you desire.

Or maybe you feel safer with NEVER and CONDITIONAL rules for everything... and prefer not to leave anything unrestricted. It's completely up to you!

However you handle your 'Unconditional' section, just be sure you remember the Pig's favorite con:

> ## "We simply MUST cheat this one time only or else we will promptly starve to death!"
> ## — Sincerely, Your Pig

Regardless of how you construct your 'Unrestricted' category you must always ensure there is enough leeway in your overall Food Plan so you'll have enough to eat. Otherwise the Pig's Squeals start to sound more alluring — and you must always be able to dismiss them outright.

Humans evolved during times of intermittent famine. Our bodies are set up to go for long periods without eating. It takes a minimum of several weeks without food for most people to starve to death. What are the odds you're going to die if you skip a meal? Slim to none!

There's NEVER a good reason to Binge.

The Pig is NOT trying to take care of you by suggesting you'll starve if you don't make an exception to your Food Plan. Its purpose is NOT to nourish your body but to destroy your Plan so it can go on an all-out Food Orgy.

Cage the Pig and keep it there!

Conditional

There are some foods and drinks that might work for you only in certain situations, at certain times, or when accompanying certain behaviors.

Maybe you only allow yourself sports drinks after a certain amount of exercise on a given calendar day.

Maybe you get to have a certain treasured meal only when dining out with friends, but no more than twice a week.

Maybe it's that you only eat chocolate on Saturdays.

Or maybe you just eat pretzels on days when you take your son or daughter to a major league baseball game.

The point of the 'Conditional' category is to acknowledge certain foods, drinks, and food behaviors are only troublesome when left unregulated — *or only in certain situations.*

The limit on the conditions you impose only stems from your own imagination and experience. I'm not necessarily suggesting any of the examples above are good or bad. But I will leave you with one caution: Avoid letting your 'Conditional' section become *too* complex. It's very difficult to remember complex rules when you're hungry, so the simpler the better.

Keep going over your conditions until they're expressed in the simplest possible language.

Fewer, clearer rules tend to work best.

For some people this is just a sentence or two, for others it's a whole page. Still others will have NO food or drink as 'Conditional' whatsoever.

The point is to go through the exercise and think through which foods, drinks, and food behaviors you don't need to give up entirely, but which still require *some* degree of control. It can also help articulate in writing your rationale for each of these conditions to ensure the Pig is not sneaking in some Squeal.

Last, if you find you're repeatedly struggling to find the right condition for a particular food, drink, or behavior, the odds are you'd do better putting it into the 'Never' section. *(This paragraph can save you years of painful struggle so you might want to re-read it)*

There you have it.

Never, Always, Unrestricted, and Conditional.

Four beautifully simple categories to create your own personal, self-contained legal system for governing your eating from here on.

Go ahead and create a first draft of your Food Plan. Or—*for many if not the majority of people*—just ONE Food Rule to begin with which covers your single worst trigger and/or eating behavior. But before you finalize it, let me expose you to some of the most violent Squeals you're likely to hear once you've set it down in black and white.

See, your Pig absolutely hates the idea of a crystal clear Food Plan. It wants you to believe such a Plan will restrict your freedom. *But exactly the opposite is true.* Just as most great jazz players practice their scales for years before they can freely express their creative genius, so too will you need structure around food to truly enjoy not only your food, but ALL the freedom life has to offer:

THE QUESTION IS, WHO WILL BE FREE, YOU OR THE PIG?

The question isn't whether you'll have freedom of choice vs becoming enslaved to a Food Plan. The question is, will you choose to live your life as a slave to the Pig's impulses and demands, or put the animal in its cage so you can exercise your human freedom?

Besides, you already have a Food Plan whether you write it down or not! It's impossible to function each day without making decisions about what you'll never, always, sometimes, and conditionally eat. The problem is, most people make these decisions *unconsciously.*

For example, everyone *always* stops overeating at a certain point, even if that point is unhealthy. They might eat a whole pizza, but not five. And they certainly don't eat the box the pizza came in.

Almost everyone also *always* has their favorite treats too— consumed in just the right combinations and amounts.

And there are at least some things most people avoid entirely for reasons of taste, convenience, or health.

Since you already DO have a Food Plan, I'm only suggesting you take control. Make it conscious and evaluate it with the full force of your intellect. Write the darn thing down!

WARNING – DON'T CREATE AN OVERLY RESTRICTIVE FOOD PLAN

Some people confuse my emphasis on clarity, focus, and written, unbreakable Food Rules with the kind of restriction which can stimulate bulimia and/or anorexia. This is not my intention at all.

There are two ways in which restrictive eating may lead to problem, and it's important you consider them both before creating your Food Plan...

The first is restricting the amount of calories you consume to such a degree you become constantly hungry. When you're constantly hungry, the Pig Squeals become more and more powerful and many people eventually break down and Binge. That's why I STRONGLY ADVISE AGAINST severely restricting your calorie intake. It's better to first create rules that are easy to follow. This allows you to eliminate the binging and overeating behavior. Then, once you're confident in your ability to control the pig, you can "go on a diet" and eliminate some of your caloric intake – but again – the best way to do this is in moderation.

The second way restrictive eating can be harmful is if you have previously been diagnosed with an eating disorder such as anorexia or bulimia, and/or if you've used restrictive eating in the past as a tool to avoid eating altogether and/or to avoid eating nutritionally important types of foods.

If you've been diagnosed with an eating disorder and/or have used restrictive eating before to drastically reduce your caloric intake beyond safe levels, then you should be very careful about creating eating rules. It does not mean that you can't use the Never Binge

Again method, because after all, everyone needs a Food Plan. However in this case I advise you only create rules with the help of a psychologist/psychiatrist and a dietician so you do not fall into the trap of abusing the food rules as you've done in the past.

However... if you are confident in your ability to create a healthy Food Plan which provides your body enough calories and nutrition—*and your only real concern is your ability to stick to it*—then by all means, please proceed!

Now, I've purposefully avoided recommending any particular Food Plan and/or positioning myself as a dietary or nutritional expert because the moment I even hint at telling you what to eat, your Pig will inevitably Squeal "We could NEVER eat like that! You might as well stop right here"

See, your Pig would LOVE to turn this into a big nutritional debate because there's still a lot of controversy about what constitutes the ideal diet. And the Pig knows that immersing you in this controversy would distract you from the main point, which is permanently committing to a Food Plan of *your own* design, using *your own* best thinking.

But now you're aware of this Pig strategy, so you won't be vulnerable to it...

FREE STARTER TEMPLATES FOR
YOUR PERSONAL FOOD PLAN

Find a great starting point no matter what you personally believe is the healthiest way to eat! The templates are part of the FREE book bonuses available on the website. When you download them you'll also find a Custom Food Plan Worksheet to take you through the creation of your own plan in much more detail.

Click Here Now to Download:
www.NeverBingeAgain.com

Now, believe it or not if you've read this far, you've actually got enough information in your brain to defeat your fat-thinking-self forever:

> ➢ The Pig is NOT You. It is a conceptual, animalistic entity which misdirects your survival drive towards food behaviors that do NOT serve your best interests, and causes you to keep changing your mind about your commitments. Unfortunately, due to our anatomy we're all forced to spend a lifetime with this presence inside. But we *can* choose to intellectually and emotionally sever it from our own definition of self. In so doing we separate from the onslaught of destructive urges and irrational thinking to which we were previously vulnerable. We can stop behaving against our own best judgment and pursue our goals and aspirations *without* ongoing sabotage. We will lock the Pig in a cage and dominate it completely, showing it nothing but contempt. Many years of suffering have proven it will dominate *us* if we do anything else.

> ➢ To accomplish this, you must take 100% responsibility for defining your own unambiguous Food Plan. You can draw inspiration from various experts and books, but nobody — *not even the most renowned diet expert* — can follow you around to be sure you comply. For this reason, and because nobody knows how your body reacts as well as you do, the buck absolutely must stop with you. There are free starter templates available on the website.

> ➢ Define your Food Plan with 100% clarity so you can tell with certainty when you are ON versus OFF it.

> ➢ A Binge = even one bite and/or swallow outside of your Food Plan.

> ➢ You will NEVER Binge again.

> Pig Squeal *(fat thinking)* is ANY thought, feeling, or impulse which suggests you may ever even consider the possibility of Bingeing again. Since you *(your thin-thinking-self)* will NEVER do it — *and since there's just you and the Pig inside your head* — anything which even remotely suggests you will do otherwise must be coming from the Pig.

> Pig Slop is anything which violates your Food Plan even 0.00001%. Bingeing = putting even the tiniest bit of Pig Slop in your mouth.

> Your Pig's Trough is where its Slop belongs. You never eat out of a Pig's Trough, so you will never eat Pig Slop again.

> From now on when the Pig Squeals for its Slop, you will just ignore it. Only Pigs eat Slop and you are not a Pig, so there's never any reason to engage or debate the Pig about the idea.

> In this way, you may defeat the Pig forever.

Even though the above is all you need to dominate your Pig, it will work hard to sneak Squeals past you in every possible manner. So let's review some of the most alluring Squeals you're likely to hear once you resolve to dominate the Pig. For example, your Pig may already be saying something like:

"Glenn says you'll be weak and vulnerable until you've heard all of my best techniques. That means we can keep on Bingeing until you finish this book! Take your time because it's Yummy!!! Yipppeeeee!!!!"
– Sincerely, Your Pig

See what I mean?

What a Pig!

But still, in much the same way prisoners of war can be inoculated against brainwashing by pre-exposing them to the techniques their captors are likely to use, you can benefit from the accumulated wisdom of those who've defeated their own Pigs before you.

For this reason — *and even though NONE of the Pig's Squeals ever stand up to the light of reason* — we will address and dispel your Pig's sneakiest Squeals as we progress.

In other words, I'll prepare you with foreknowledge of the many stupid, stupid ways the Pig will try to trick you.

Not surprisingly, the very first thing your Pig may say after you've sworn your sacred oath to your Food Plan is "You're just being silly now. How will you manage those inevitable, irresistible cravings?"

CHAPTER 2

How to 'Deal' with Cravings

First of all...

You do not have cravings – your pig does! So when you feel one coming on, just say:

"I WILL NEVER EAT PIG SLOP AGAIN!"

(Then move on to a more valuable way to spend your time and energy, or a healthier way to nourish your body, mind, and soul)

From where you sit right now, it might be hard to believe this is ALL you need for dominating any craving. But it's true. In fact, the conclusion flows naturally from the definition of the Pig itself:

THREE STEPS TO DEFEAT ANY CRAVING

1. **Remember:** Consuming even the most minuscule amount of Pig Slop —*anything even remotely off of your well defined Food Plan*—is, by definition, a Binge.

2. **Recall:** All thoughts and feelings which suggest you may ever Binge again are Pig Squeal. Therefore *you* do not have cravings, your Pig does. ALL cravings are Pig Squeal.

3. **Reiterate:** So just quietly but proudly say to yourself[1] "I will never eat Pig Slop again!" *(Some people like to add "And I shall remain 100% committed to my Food Plan until my dying breath")* Then go on with your day, ignoring the Squeals.

That's all.

Or you can just use the shorthand:

"That's Pig Slop, and I NEVER eat Pig Slop!"

You might want to print this out and carry it around for a while.

Oh wait... did you hear that? Your Pig just got very excited:

"Glenn says to Never Binge Again you need to carry around these three steps. That means if you ever forget them — *which you know you will* — we can just Binge until you remember. Yummmmmy!!!" — Sincerely, Your Pig

What a Pig!

Just remember ONE thing and you'll be fine:

---

[1]   IMPORTANT: Your Food Plan is a very private and personal matter. Other people's Food Plans are not really any of your business unless you're invited to discuss them. Telling someone else they're eating Pig Slop is a great way to ruin a perfectly good relationship. Everyone gets to decide what goes in their Pig's trough vs what goes on their personal human plate. In fact, everyone gets to decide for themselves whether they want to separate their fat thinking self *(the Pig)* from their thin-thinking-self *at all.* You've therefore got NO real way of knowing how to define Pig Slop for anyone but yourself! More on this in the chapter on dealing with other people's Pigs.

You Will Never Eat Pig Slop Again!

By definition, every craving is nothing more than a desire for Pig Slop — every last one. So just ignore it and go on with your life.

Let's make it even simpler: The one and only thing you need to do to ensure you do not Binge is 'not Binge!' Mind blowing, isn't it? Still, some people find it comforting to carry around the above three-step reminder. Enough said.

Now, other people tell me that even though they understand and agree with the definitions above, the cravings are too uncomfortable to tolerate. These people don't realize the Pig has convinced them of yet another insane proposition: That one must be comfortable at all times, and that Bingeing is the ONLY way to alleviate discomfort.

Unfortunately, we all must share our bodies with our Pigs. So, when the Pig has cravings, we indeed might feel uncomfortable — if we haven't taken a few precautions first. Sometimes even if we have.

Momentarily I'll tell you how to eliminate *most* of this discomfort, but one critical point first:

YOU DO NOT NEED TO BE COMFORTABLE TO STICK TO YOUR FOOD PLAN *(FOREVER!)*

Because the Pig is a survival drive run amuck, it thinks it will literally die without comfort. This is why it will go to any length to get you to feed it. But comfort is not a "must have," only a "nice to have." Therefore, before your Pig will let up, it will need to know you're willing to tolerate ANY level of discomfort without Bingeing.

Of course, feeling bad for the sake of feeling bad would be masochistic, so we will definitely take steps to make ourselves comfortable. But if we're going to hold our Food Plans sacred, there *will* be times we feel uncomfortable. So be it. Our Pigs must know we will NEVER consider these times Bingeing opportunities.

45

Let's do a little thought experiment to illustrate your in-born ability to tolerate enough discomfort to Never Binge Again. First, bring to mind some Slop your Pig would absolutely love to eat — its favorite junk.

Next, think of someone you love dearly — perhaps your son or your daughter, or maybe a spouse, sibling, parent, or beloved pet. *(If there's nobody in your life you love dearly right now, think of a role model or celebrity you care about.)*

Before you go any further, please be sure you really are thinking of a special person — AND — something your Pig craves with all of its gluttonous essence. This exercise will only take a few moments, but you'll remember it the rest of your life. It can dramatically strengthen your ability to manage cravings, so don't let your Pig cheat you out of it by suggesting you skip this, OK?

OK!

Now assume an evil dictator is stalking the person you picked, and he presents you with a twisted choice: Although he will continue watching your special person forever, the dictator will never contact, influence, or harm them in any way — *provided you abstain from the Pig Slop under consideration until you draw your very last breath.*

But if you ever indulge again — *no matter how far in the future, no matter how small the amount, and no matter what the circumstance* — the evil dictator will kidnap and hold them in a prison for the rest of their lives. You'll always know the one indulgence you just "couldn't resist" was solely responsible for depriving your very special person of their freedom forevermore.

Remember, this dictator has the resources of an entire country behind him, so the authorities are powerless to stop him. The ONLY way to keep your special person safe is to completely abstain from even one more bite or swallow of your Pig's favorite Slop — *forever.* You'll literally have to avoid it for the rest of your life as if it were poison because the consequences are so grave.

What would you do?

It's a no-brainer, isn't it?

When you care enough, tolerating any level of discomfort FOREVER is suddenly within your power. No matter how strong a craving the Pig might throw at you.

No matter how much the Pig may Squeal for its junk, I've got little doubt you'd keep your word in this situation.

Your Pig needs to know this! It must understand you're willing to tolerate any level of discomfort without ever Bingeing again. This does not mean you *must* feel uncomfortable, just that if you do, so be it.

With this key distinction between the desirability and necessity of comfort behind us, let's talk about what you can actually do to make yourself more comfortable while you cage the Pig.

The key is recognizing there is a very real survival drive which the Pig hijacks and turns against us. Humans are wired to seek sustenance as a major priority in three situations: (1) when nutrients are depleted; (2) when we get too cold and; (3) when our blood sugar drops too low. Sometimes, we also confuse dehydration with hunger. Therefore:

You can keep the discomfort associated with cravings to a minimum by staying relatively warm and hydrated, and consuming regular, consistent, healthy meals.

Most people can almost totally eliminate the physiological experience of cravings when they attend to these elements of self-care.

There's one more very important thing you can do to ward off cravings: Acknowledge the difference between killing a craving and "getting high" with the hyper-palatable treats our modern food industry has engineered to overstimulate our brain's reward centers. Your Pig wants to get high with food, but your goal is *only* to eliminate the craving so you can go on with your day.

Perhaps the concept of getting high with food is new to you. That wouldn't surprise me because our culture actually condones and reinforces the habit. It doesn't identify the experience for what it really is.

Economic incentives have sent the industry on a never-ending quest to make foods which push our evolutionary buttons — foods with high caloric density, and foods with progressively more addictive potential. Unfortunately this pursuit is so lucrative, things will probably only get worse in our lifetimes. It's unfortunately very difficult to stop a giant economic machine.

This likely is not news to you.

What most people don't realize, however, is WHY our economic infrastructure developed to support this type of activity in the first place. And, if we're going to have a more mature attitude about food — *and make the Pig's Squeals even less alluring* —it's helpful to understand how these forces developed. Knowledge is power.

The very fabric of society once depended on its ability to refine food in this unnatural way. When it became necessary for larger tribes to send armies over longer distances, it was difficult to transport enough whole, natural food to feed the soldiers on the journey. And as our society developed specialization of labor, we required workers to spend whole days focused on their singular trade, rather than hunting and gathering for themselves.

This is why ultra-dense, portable sources of calories became an essential part of our civil structure. In many ways — *though there are now much better alternatives available* — the survival and economic balance of nations once depended on these foods, and they've become firmly entrenched in our culture.

Beyond this, the prevalence of disease before modern medicine made being too thin much more of a risk than being too fat. And only recently have most societies become able to keep starvation at bay for a majority of the population.

These are among many of the stronger reasons it became a moral transgression to waste food in our society. And why just a few hundred years ago in Europe, being portly or chubby was a sign of higher status, as was the "luxury" of consuming white flour, and white sugar!

These forces—*in addition to the ridiculously delicious nature of those super-rewarding foods heavy in sugar, salt, and oil, etc.*— caused us to develop cooking habits and social norms to ensure continued demand. For anyone to eat in another manner was a threat to society itself. The offender need either be reined in or cast out!

Moreover, "reining in" back then was much different than we think of it now. Today, acting differently than society as a whole is acceptable and even encouraged to a certain extent. But in the old days individualism was very dangerous because it threatened the survival of the tribe. While today you'll only be made to *feel* like an outcast if you eat differently than everyone else, back then it was more like "step out of line and we'll kill you!" There was only a certain amount of food available, of a certain kind, at a particular time. So you ate what everyone else ate or you died. Period.

And even though things may be a *little* better now thanks to the healthy foods movement, there's still a very strongly enculturated preference for gluttony *("Supersize that please")* which is aided and abetted by big Agriculture with its nutritional denials and GMO modifications, not to mention the profits of big Pharma which treats the resulting diseases.

This is how our Pigs became fortified with (1) the extremely pleasurable drive to consume super-rewarding, ultra-processed foods *(the "Food High")*; (2) very strong social and familial support for indulgence; (3) traditions and Holidays which reinforce the use of these foods; (4) unspoken cultural prohibitions against abstaining; (5) the unspoken threat of becoming an outcast if you eat differently than the rest of society.

In short, our society actually WANTS you to get high with food. The world around you is mostly on your Pig's side. To defeat the Pig, you must become willing to face this situation. *(Once you do, it's easy!)*

The situation food abusers face today is very different than that faced by people who choose other substances. When a substance abuser indulges, they're making a choice to act _against_ societal pressures and norms. When they stop, they fall back into line with cultural norms, and more easily integrate into society.

The exact opposite is true with food.

Food abusers are actually supported by our culture to continue eating poorly. To get healthier, they must make a choice to act *against* societal pressures and norms. To *stop* abusing food means embracing *more* unease and conflict with others. There are fewer restaurants you can easily eat in. Fewer markets to shop in. Family and friends will pressure you to eat the way they do. I could go on and on.

Thankfully there *is* a growing community of healthy eaters where people who wish to stop getting high with food may find refuge. You can dominate the Pig regardless of social pressure as long as you know what's going on around you.

You can and will also learn to recognize the Pig Squeal stimulated by other people's Pigs and the food industry as a whole—even when nobody else acknowledges what's happening. All great progress begins with one person's willingness to stand against the crowd, and right here in this book you have all the necessary tools to do it.

In fact, it wouldn't matter if you were the only person in the world who wanted to eat healthy. As long as you're conscious of the social dilemma, you won't be fooled. Just recognize the voices of industry and culture you're surrounded by as Pig Squeal. And then remember you will never eat Pig Slop again, no matter what anyone else says!

Remember: All the Pig wants is one more Food High, and it will use the very fabric of society to back up its claims. It believes you will literally die if you don't Binge on some Slop, pronto!

But the Pig is wrong.

When you stick to your Food Plan and nourish your body you will NOT die.

But you won't get a Food High either.

You'll just kill the Craving and go on with your day.

This will NOT be exhilarating.

You'll experience life however life was meant to be on that particular day without a food high...

But YOU will be 100% in control.

This is the only way to get the results you want.

Killing a Craving is like pouring water on a fire in your back yard so you don't burn down the house. Getting high with food is like throwing gasoline on the fire and inhaling the fumes.

When you kill the Craving you're left with a few carefully contained, smoldering ashes which eventually die out on their own accord. But if you inhale the fumes, you'll obtain a brief sense of euphoria before being left with a much bigger problem to manage.

Another helpful analogy is contentment *(killing the Craving)* vs. mania *(the Food High)*. Contentment is a gentle state of mind available to anyone who seeks it. It's not something people feel compelled to get up on the rooftops and shout about. Contentment is a solid, repeatable state which builds sustainable confidence, and a rational and responsible sense of well-being.

51

Mania, on the other hand, is inherently unstable. The Pig knows the Food High will eventually wear off, so it frantically Squeals to extend the high by Bingeing "just a little" more.

Mania is an unstable, temporary pleasure which becomes progressively more difficult to repeat. Just like with drugs, the Pig will require more Slop during each subsequent Binge in order to obtain the same high it experienced previously. This is what drug addicts call "chasing the dragon", and it destroys the Binger's confidence, health, and sense of wellbeing the longer it's allowed to occur.

So how do you deal with Cravings?

Cage the Pig, man... just cage it and keep it locked up!

Your Pig has Cravings... you don't. And you will NEVER eat Pig Slop again.

Be willing to tolerate ANY level of discomfort to keep to your solemn vow—but stay nourished, warm, and hydrated to keep this to a minimum.

Kill Cravings, don't get high with food.

End of story.

FREE CRAVING DEFEATER WALLET CARD + MP3

Before we move on, if you haven't done so already please download the Craving Defeater Cheat Card and MP3 available as part of the FREE book upgrade package. Together these two pack a powerful one-two punch to neutralize the Pig when it bothers you with its Cravings. (www.NeverBingeAgain.com)

CHAPTER 3

What if You DO Binge?

The first time you make a mistake you'll almost certainly hear something like this from your Pig:

> "You cheated! You cheated! You cheated!!! See? Your Food Plan doesn't mean anything at all! The Hell with this *'Never Binge Again!'* stuff. You'll have to try something else to control me. YOU'VE BLOWN IT SO I AM NOW TOTALLY FREE TO BINGE AT WILL FROM NOW ON!!! Yippeeee!!! Yippeeee!!! Party Time!!! Let's Do It!!!!"
> – Your Pig

This one Squeal causes more damage than virtually any other because it allows a small Binge to snowball into a full-blown Food Orgy, and seriously undermines confidence in your ability to control yourself.

This Squeal is wholly responsible for the "Screw it, you already blew it, just start again tomorrow" mentality. Or, in shorthand, the "F___ It" Squeal.

Learning to recognize and ignore the F__ It Squeal is, without a doubt, the most significant benefit of the Never Binge Again approach.

Thankfully this Squeal, like every other, is easily defeated once you see it for what it is. But because our culture actually supports Binge thinking, it can be hard to identify.

For example, I'm sure you've heard the idea of "progress, not perfection" bandied about by the so called experts. They may even quote scientific evidence which suggests perfectionism is a set up for a Binge.

While these are alluring ideas which can be helpful when placed in context, they unfortunately only tell HALF the story. What these half-truths fail to acknowledge is the significant difference in attitude required _before_ vs. _after_ a food mistake. Just like we can't walk on water or swim on dry land, we must maneuver very differently before vs. after a Binge. *(Remember, a Binge is even one bite or swallow outside of your very well defined Food Plan)*:

> **BEFORE A BINGE:** Your Food Plan is 100% perfect and final. You Will NEVER Make a Mistake Again. You Will NEVER Binge Again!

> **AFTER A BINGE:** You are a fallible human being. You were *practicing* a set of Food Rules, but that practice is now over and it's time for the big leagues. Analyze what went wrong, adjust your Food Plan if necessary, and THEN declare it perfect and final. You may have found it necessary to divorce the old Food Plan *(or simply failed to hear the Pig's Squeals about it)*, but now you're a changed person, ready to marry once again. You Will NEVER Binge Again!

The Pig wants to confuse these two situations so you'll reject your Food Plan as nonsensical. Why? So it can Binge of course!

I hope you're starting to see a pattern. Bingeing is ALL the Pig ever wants, and there's NEVER a reason to listen to it before, during, or after a mistake.

The Pig's "confuse and conquer" maneuver is easily defeated when you place your thinking in the right context.

WHY PERFECTION IS THE BEST COMMITMENT TOOL: Making a sacred commitment to your Food Plan is like getting married. And I've yet to hear these vows at a wedding ceremony:

> *"I promise to love and be faithful...until an inevitable moment of weakness. I promise I'll do the best I can, but nobody's perfect and there sure are a lot of attractive people out there. I'm 80% sure I can be faithful forever, but anyone who promises you 100% is an unrealistic liar. A 'pretty good' promise is the best anyone can ever hope for, because you can't possibly know who you're going to sleep with next year, or in ten years. Just being honest. You want me to be honest, right?" – **The Vow Your Pig Would Make at Its Wedding!**

You'd never accept this kind of a wishy-washy promise from a mate...so why entertain it for your own commitments? Your Pig craves uncertainty, not you. It will exploit even the most miniscule crisis of confidence to tear at the very fabric of your most sacred vows.

Time for another thought experiment: Suppose your fiancé—*after realizing you wouldn't accept this level of uncertainty in the wedding vows*—increased their confidence in a lifetime of fidelity from 80% to 90%. Would you marry them then?

What about 95%?

99%?

Kind of ruins the romance, doesn't it!

You wouldn't accept anything less than a 100% commitment, because perfection is the essence of commitment...all notions of human frailty aside.

PERFECTION IS ESSENCE OF COMMITMENT

Allowing ANY possibility you will ever Binge again changes the commitment from "I will" to "I'll try"...which is NO

commitment at all. <u>The "little engine that could" was in error</u>. "I think I can" is the wrong philosophy. "I know I can" is the only attitude which succeeds with impulse control because your Pig will use "I'll try" to destroy the very fabric of your Food Plan.

Anything less than a plan for 100% adherence to your Food Plan is nothing more than the Pig's plan to Binge. You must authoritatively declare your Food Plan as 100% perfect or you are not committing to anything at all.

The philosophy behind "progress not perfection" as a *before* tool is one of hopeless abandon to the Pig's impulses. To adopt the "progress not perfection" ideology is to believe it's literally impossible to dominate your Cravings.

Progress-not-perfection says there will eventually come an irresistible urge which forces you to indulge... it's just a matter of time.

Cravings are indeed a natural part of being alive. You can't escape them, but once you've drawn your perfect lines in the sand you need not fear them either!

Now, there actually IS scientific evidence that perfectionism is a set up for a Binge, but what's missing from this analysis is context. Perfectionism is *only* a set up for a Binge when you allow the Pig to use it to retrospectively assign powerlessness to you—*AFTER* a mistake has occurred:

> *"Either you're perfect or you're nothing. Either you can perfectly control your food intake or you can't control it at all. You made a mistake and are therefore not perfect. Obviously, you are now completely out of control. I get to go on a big giant hairy Binge. Yippeeee!!!" - Your Pig*

Perfectionism may be a set up for a Binge when you apply it after a mistake has occurred, but when you use it to lock in your commitments at the outset just the opposite is true. Perfectionism is the right approach to gain control of your eating forever when used as a commitment tool. In fact in this context I'd contend it is the ONLY approach that works. However, when applied as a post-Binge analysis tool it works in the Pig's best interest, not yours.

To Never Binge Again and permanently stick to our commitments we must recognize any and all insecurity as 100% Pig Squeal. By definition, it can't be any other way because Pig Squeal is any thought, feeling, or impulse which suggests you will *ever* Binge again.

By definition, any and all doubt about your commitment to Never Binge Again is Pig Squeal.

Now, what if you DO Binge? Can you feel how excited your Pig is getting about the fact I'm even bothering to write this?

> "See, Glenn knows we ARE going to Binge again, otherwise he'd never put this section in the book. I'm so happy!!! Let's go already. Let's just do it!!!! C'mon already!!!" – Your Pig

What if you DO Binge? What then???

Simple: Analyze what happened, adjust your sails, and then NEVER Binge again.

Why? Because the Pig must be caged, that's why!

Period, end of story.

Notwithstanding the simplicity and elegance of this instruction, many people feel the need for more direction to get back on track after a mistake. So let's talk about the right mental maneuvers to recover from a Binge.

First, please know that after a Binge your Pig will direct all its efforts to *building* upon your mistake. And just as monsters are terrified of the light of day, the Pig prefers to hide in the dark. It knows under scrutiny you will become wise to its game, so it will try to get you to casually dismiss the mistake without examination—in hopes of keeping the errors in thinking and/or problematic Food Rules from being exposed.

In short, the Pig will martial all its efforts to stop you from carefully reflecting upon what happened and instead try to direct your energy towards Bingeing more.

Knowing the Pig's post-Binge goals, the first thing to do after a Binge is remember what a serious, solemn oath committing to our Food Plan actually was. After all, your ability to stick with your own commitments is your ability to keep your word, and without your word, you don't have much. So if you find you've made a mistake you must take it *very* seriously and become willing to carefully reflect upon what went wrong.

On the other hand, creating the perfect set of Food Rules for any given individual is a complex matter... not unlike creating a set of laws to govern a large, interactive society.

Successful legal systems always contain a mechanism for self-correction. For example, although the framers of the United States Constitution fully intended it to govern as the law of the land, they understood it was still a potentially fallible document. So they included a mechanism for amending it over time.

But the process for amending the Constitution does *not* allow for impulsivity. It requires a drawn out process of proposals, votes, and ratification. These delays ensure serious consideration is given to the ramifications of change, and make it difficult for any one crazed person *(or group)* to seize power and undo all the good work.

Therefore, the first thing to do after a Binge is to examine what happened. Review your Food Plan with an eye towards determining whether you believe each Food Rule within it is still in your best interest.

Is the Food Plan as a whole still the most accurate representation of a perfect, healthy lifestyle? Or does something need to be amended?

More often than not, Binges occur simply because you failed to hear the Pig's Squeal, NOT because of a problem with the Food Plan itself. The Pig slipped in a few destructive words which you mistook for your own thinking, and you acted upon them.

This is called a "Simple Pig Attack" and requires NO changes to your Plan. If you've experienced a Simple Pig Attack just put the Pig back in its cage forever by re-committing in full to the exact Food Plan you just broke.

This is what we mean by "just Never Binge Again" as the best mechanism for fast and permanent recovery. But remember, your Pig will Squeal violently because it doesn't want to go back into its cage, once again locked away from its Slop forever. Listen for things like:

> "You obviously can't lock me in my cage forever. You're too weak. I just got out, so of course I'll get out again. Maybe I can't beat you now but it's only a matter of time until we Binge again. Yippee!!!"– *Your Pig's response upon hearing you will Never Binge Again after a recent indulgence*

This is utter Pig Squeal and has NO constructive purpose. The Pig doesn't care about your well-being at all. It ONLY wants Slop, so why would you ever take its thoughts seriously?

Just ignore the Pig on this matter, don't debate it.

Notwithstanding the above, having rational answers for this nonsense is helpful to many people as they're first learning how to cage the Pig. So let's address the Pig's "points":

> ➢ "You're too weak"à Making a renewed effort to eat more constructively is evidence of strength, not weakness. Even if you've repeatedly fallen down for years, continuing to get

up until you succeed is a mark of fortitude and perseverance, not weakness. A weak person just listens to the Pig and gives up. A strong one resolves to lock the Pig back in its cage forever. Making a renewed vow of abstinence proves your strength. When you think about it this way, you'll see how truly pathetic it is that the Pig would attempt to use your renewed vow against you!

> "I just got out, so of course I'll get out again."à It's extremely unusual for prisoners to break out of jail twice unless the jailor consciously and purposefully leaves the door open.

> "Maybe I can't beat you right now but it's only a matter of time until we Binge again."à Since you have full control over what you buy, open, take out of the package with your hands, put in your mouth, chew, and swallow, you will _always_ have the 100% ability to keep the Pig in its cage. You don't have to worry about "later", only the present, and it is always the present.

That's how to defeat the Pig after a simple Pig Attack.

But what if you believe your Food Plan itself was at fault?

For example, what if YOU (not your Pig!) believe you've erroneously committed to a Plan which is too restrictive and leaves you uncomfortably hungry and/or missing key nutrients?

If this is the case you're going to need to go ahead and change it. But before you do (a) be sure you've given yourself some time for the Pig Slop you've ingested to leave your system because it's hard to hear the Pig's Squeals when your body's full of Pig Slop; (b) Save a dated copy of your complete Food Plan before making any changes so you can roll it back later if you find the Pig has influenced the changes; (c) Take some serious, reflective time to "think on paper" about the specific changes you're planning to make; (d) Consider whether any previous version of your Food Plan was better. It's not unusual for mistakes to have occurred because the Pig convinced you to abandon a perfectly good Food Plan. If this is the case, just revert to the old one. And since you save a dated copy of every version, this is easy to do.

Here's one more thing to consider as you re-examine your Food Plan: If you find you're repeatedly struggling with a food or drink in the Conditionals section, the odds are pretty good you need to move it to the Nevers. For many people, certain super-rewarding foods taste and feel too good to constrain with conditions and rules. But these same people—*who may have struggled for years or even decades with a particular food*—find it remarkably easy to NEVER have it again. Certainly much easier than the ongoing, painful search for that one "magic rule" which will let them have their cake and eat it too.

Never can be a LOT easier than sometimes!

Last, during the "legislative process"—*the time during which you are re-examining your Food Plan*—it's best if you allow the previous rules to govern, however imperfect they may be. The Pig craves the anarchy which underlies a Binge. Therefore, under no circumstances should you ever allow "the absence of a government" to exist—even for a micro-second.

And remember, you made a mistake, you didn't have a brain operation which disabled your ability to make good food choices, or to control your hands, arms, legs, mouth, and tongue. You have not had a mysterious curse laid upon you which prevents you from eating well. Space aliens have not abducted you and implanted electrodes which force you to eat Pig Slop. Whatever new rules you may consider, you are 100% in charge of feeding yourself throughout the entire process! Finally...

After a serious analysis of what caused the mistake, promptly forgive yourself and make a 100% confident, renewed commitment to _perfectly_ follow your Food Plan forever.

You are a fallible human being. You were *practicing* a particular Food Plan, but now practice is over. It's time for the big leagues. You analyzed what went wrong, and made the necessary adjustments so...

You Will Never Binge Again!

And all you need to do to never binge again is never binge again.

You might consider reading the above sentence a few times because your Pig would very much like you to think otherwise, especially right after a Binge.

Cage the Pig and keep it there!

In the next chapter we're going to tackle and defeat a serious paradox: You must simultaneously view your Food Plan as perfect AND remain amenable to change. *(So you can grow from experience and incorporate new information as it becomes available)*

FREE BINGE RECOVERY TOOLS

Here's a strange thought: Since you will Never Binge Again you actually won't ever need these tools. And your Pig loves that they exist because they suggest the possibility you might consider feeding it. Let the Pig wallow in its Cage! All you need to do to never binge again is never binge again. Profound, isn't it?

However, because it can be a little tricky to master the two different ways of thinking required before vs. after a Binge, many people find having specific tools available for Binge recovery extremely helpful. Therefore, I've prepared a free workbook and accompanying MP3 for your smart phone to walk you through the re-establishment of your commitment—and more importantly your confidence!—after a Binge has occurred.

It's part of the FREE book upgrade available at www. NeverBingeAgain.com

CHAPTER 4

Is Just One Bite Off
Your Food Plan REALLY a Binge?

I take a LOT of heat for defining a Binge as just one bite off your carefully defined Food Plan. The critics say it's an impossible standard and I'm just setting people up for a Binge when they fail to meet it.

But I emphatically disagree.

See, this line of thinking assumes one MUST go on an all-out food orgy the moment one realizes a mistake's been made...

When the more intelligent thing to do at that juncture is recognize "We already blew it so we might as well just Binge our faces off for the rest of the day" as a big hairy Pig Squeal in and of itself...

And just put the Pig back in its Cage and resume...

No matter what happened five seconds, five minutes, five months, or five years ago!

As reviewed previously, there's no reason to bang all your teeth out with a hammer the moment you realize you've chipped a tooth...

No reason for an archer to shoot all the rest of his *(or her)* arrows off to the side of the target just because they missed the bulls eye once ...

And no reason to repeatedly touch a hot stove because you accidently burned yourself once!

Always use the present moment to be healthy...and you'll be fine.

Without the "one bite off your Food Plan is a Binge" criteria, your personal Food Bullseye will become fuzzy and vague...

And if you don't know where the target is, how in the world are you going to hit it?

My critics would have me tell you to just kinda-sorta aim in the direction of the target... but that makes it MUCH more likely you're going to miss when compared to a target you can actually SEE with crystal clarity?

Why not draw clear boundaries around the bullseye so you can concentrate all your energy—*indeed the very essence of your being*—on hitting it?

Then if you happen to miss, just analyze, readjust and commit once again. If you keep doing this your aim MUST get better...

But not if you're prevented from aiming in the first place. And that's what the "fuzzy target" philosophy *("progress not perfection" and "guidelines rather than rules")* does to us...

It prevents us from aiming in EXACTLY the right direction!

Well, I don't know about you, but if the game's going to be rigged against me from the outset I'd rather just sit still and repeatedly smack myself in the head with a spatula.

But screw that noise, man...

Because I'm NOT going to be visiting the emergency room any time soon with deep spatula wounds ...

I'm going to aim at MY personal Food Bullseye...

And I'm going to know EXACTLY where it is.

If I screw up, I'm just going to recommit again...

Because that's the ONLY way I've ever found to purge all the doubt and insecurity from my mind so I can concentrate on the goal.

My Pig HATES this plan...

But it gives ME tremendous confidence...

And if one of us has to suffer, well, you know which one it's going to be!

One bite off of your carefully defined Food Plan IS a Binge...

But the moment you realize you've done it you just stop and get right back on track. "We're off the Plan so let's have a Binging Party" is pure Pig Squeal to be ignored...

Plus... if you don't take the first bite, this is all a moot point.

There is a valid reason to differentiate small mistakes from all-out-food-orgies, however, as you are analyzing your progress. Even though you can Never Binge Again... the practical course most people follow involves falling down and getting up several times.

In this light, it's helpful to be able to look back and say "I'm catching the Binges sooner and doing a lot less damage with them." Indeed the first thing most people notice is the disappearance of All Out Food Orgies.

So if you'd like to distinguish between a "slip" stepping off your Food Plan by just a few bites vs. an All Out Food Orgy involving thousands of calories and a general "Pig run rampant"... be my guest.

But whatever you do, don't blur the line between being on vs. off your Food Plan because you'll be creating a hole your Pig can run right through. And if your Food Plan is too restrictive, change it!

CHAPTER 5

Changing Your Food Plan

There's a big Paradox inherent in the idea of changing our Food Plan. On the one hand, to have *any* chance of success we must 100% commit to the plan we swore at the outset. Otherwise the Pig will be able to tear the tiny hole we're leaving in the fabric of our Plan wide open, and burst out into a big giant Food Orgy.

On the other hand, experimentation and learning are the underpinning of all progress. We must always integrate new evidence as it becomes available. And we must be able to learn from our mistakes. The best Food Plans *evolve* over time, so it's critical to retain the ability to adapt.

For example, a few weeks ago my doctor brought a new series of studies to my attention which suggested fruit is metabolized *faster* in the presence of fatty foods, not slower as was previously thought. This meant my "only eat fruit with nuts and seeds" rule—*which was originally intended to keep my glycemic load down and manage my genetic predisposition to high triglycerides*—was actually counterproductive. It would be foolhardy to insist on sticking to this rule in the context of this new information, even though I'd previously committed 100%.

Similarly, because the food industry spends billions on developing cheap, super-rewarding foods—*and very persuasive packaging*—many people are unwilling to put certain types of Pig Slop in their Pig's trough vs. their human plates. Their Pig begs and pleads to keep its Slop in the Conditionals section of the Food Plan, putting forth endless variations of rules it says it will follow *"this time"*... if we'll only give it one more chance.

Our natural inclination is to leave as much pleasure in our diets as possible. And because a good Food Plan should indeed also be pleasurable, it can take several rounds of experimentation to weed out the Pig's impulses for *toxic* pleasure from your own innate healthy desires.

Upon Serious Reflection You May Change Your Food Plan At Any Time...*But Your Pig Never Will Again!!*

We must adapt our Food Plan when the reasons are sound—even though each time we commit to it we have every intention of NEVER changing it again. But because the Pig will always do everything in its power to convince us Bingeing is perfectly rational, we must apply a simple procedure to ensure the changes are not Pig driven. So it's important to ask yourself these challenge questions before changing your Food Plan:

> ➤ Have you made a written copy of your existing Food Plan and saved it somewhere you can easily retrieve in case you need to "roll back" to your best previous plan? The Pig seeks anarchy so it can Binge. Saving and protecting "the law" in the event a repeal becomes necessary is something *people* do, not Pigs.

> ➤ Have you taken the time to "think on paper" about your proposed change? Your Pig will insist most changes it desires are extremely urgent because it knows you're unlikely to decide in its favor if you think too much about what's being proposed. People treat changes to the law as serious matters worthy of careful reflection and analysis. Pigs want immediate change for immediate pleasure. People use their intellect and delay-of-gratification abilities to make wiser, healthier choices.

➢ Are you being very specific about the change itself? Generally speaking, Food Plans improve slowly and specifically over time *(like the law)*. But Pigs argue for vaguely articulated changes which are often sweeping and impulsive in nature.

➢ Can you articulate the detailed and specific *reason* behind the change you wish to make? *(Not the change itself, but the reason for it)*.Poorly articulated reasons for change are more likely to be Pig driven. The Pig's primary rationale is "because it will taste/feel good." Because this reason is so primitive and transparent, the Pig prefers it not be articulated at all. So before changing your plan, ask yourself if the change you are contemplating represents a legitimate opportunity to improve your nutrition, comfort level, and well-being. Articulate the reason YOU believe this in detail, and then analyze that reason just to be sure no Pig Squeal has snuck in.

➢ Are you sure any change is necessary at all? Most often the reason for a Binge is a simple Pig Attack *(unrecognized Pig Squeal)*, not a problem with the Food Plan itself. But the emotions and physiological disturbances associated with Bingeing can make us FEEL like something's horribly wrong which must change immediately. Would it be more constructive to just resume and 100% re-commit to your Food Plan as is?

➢ If the change under consideration was prompted by having Binged, has enough TIME passed for your body to rid itself of the physical influence of Pig Slop? This can require few days. In the interim you can't trust your biological hunger mechanisms... they've been temporarily corrupted by the Pig. You must take particular care to make *intellectually* sound food choices after a Binge.

➢ Even if the change under consideration was NOT prompted by a Binge, have you given at least a few day's consideration to all the above?

If you can get through the above questions successfully, then it's almost certainly YOU who are making the change, not your Pig, and you should go forward once again with 100% confidence.

It's perfectly fine to change your Food Plan as long as you're sure YOU are doing it for good reason, and are not under the influence of the Pig. Moreover, notwithstanding the seeming Big Paradox, we must be able and willing to adapt as we learn.

Just use the challenge questions above to be sure it's YOU who's doing the adapting and not your Pig! *(Note: For a printable one-sheet you can hang on your wall with these criteria, please download the "How to Change Your Food Plan" cheat sheet at* www. NeverBingeAgain.com*)*

CHAPTER 6

The Time Counting Trap

Our culture emphasizes counting time to address addiction. Just as alcoholics are encouraged to remember exactly how long it's been since their last drink, people who love food may be tempted to keep track of the last time they Binged.

While there IS definitely merit in keeping track of streaks for the first 90 days or so to help establish new habits, it's a serious mistake in my not-so-humble opinion to seek public recognition for it.

Here's why...

Publicly counting the number of days, months, or years it's been since you last Binged is like shouting out the length of time you've been obeying the law in the public square. In our society the law is the law and we simply expect people to comply—*we don't give them a medal when they do!*

Try this thought experiment: Imagine someone proclaiming "it's been three weeks since I ran a red light" or "it's been a whole year since I robbed a bank" and you'll see just how ridiculous public time counting can become.

Unfortunately, this practice is more than just a silly game—it's actually harmful because it signals the Pig you are insecure and ambivalent about your commitment. Worse yet, it orients your entire social identity squarely around your food problems, rather than your aspirations, abilities, and dreams.

Just like there's no reason to publicly declare how long it's been since you last ran a red light, there's NO reason to publicly declare the number of days since you last Binged.

Medals and public recognition are not given out for how long you've obeyed the law. Obeying is just the price you're expected to pay for societal privileges—not the least of which include your freedom.

Publicly counting time is the Pig's way of orienting your whole social life around Pig Slop... and setting you up for humiliation *(and an associated Binge to "make you feel better")* whenever you might make a mistake.

Publicly counting time reinforces the idea your ability to remain Binge-free is somehow linked to what other people think of you... when what you want is a sense of independent confidence in your ability to control this thing FOR LIFE.

Beyond this, counting time beyond 90 days tells your Pig that sooner or later you will "collapse under the weight of all these days." In contrast, when something's been installed in your character as a lifelong habit, you'll do it effortlessly without having to think of how long it's been. So be 100% clear with your Pig: This is a life-long arrangement and you will Never Binge Again. Otherwise, you'll just be giving it a calendar to mark off the days in hopes of one day being released.

The Pig does not deserve a calendar.

The Pig had plenty of time to prove itself a worthy citizen during the years you were open to listening to it. All it did with this privilege was try to ruin your best laid plans, goals, and dreams.

Let the Pig stay in its cage of toxic desires and unsatisfactory rewards forever!

You won't be getting up in the town square seeking recognition for how long it's been since you've run a red light. There's no "clock" to pin on yourself as a medal for public recognition.

Your Pig may want to define your whole life according to its last taste of Pig Slop, but compliance with your Food Plan is a normal and expected part of citizenship in your more objective, balanced, and respectful view of yourself. It's not something to be lauded and applauded in public. Deriving self-worth from other peoples' recognition of your compliance stacks the deck in the Pig's favor because the moment you make a mistake it can say:

> "You made a mistake and now you're going to lose ALL the public recognition you've worked so hard to obtain. Oh well, no use crying over spilled milk. Sure, you've lost face in the public's eye, but there's still ONE great thing we can do, right? Let's Binge Binge Binge Binge Binge!!! You're going to have to start over tomorrow anyway, so you might as well set me free. Yippee!!!" – Sincerely, Your Pig

This is why your Food Plan and how long you've been on it is nobody's business but your own. You've made a permanent decision to become a law-abiding, non-Bingeing citizen.

One more thought experiment to drive home the point: Suppose you run a red light. Does this give you license to blaze through every subsequent one? Of course not!

Society expects you to stop at every red light no matter what you did at the last one. You're not excused from the responsibility of obeying normal traffic laws because you have some "red light running disease." **Making a mistake doesn't invalidate the law.** Your Food Plan remains law at every possible moment in time, no matter what no matter what no matter what.

The law is the law and your Pig will just have to live with that. Forever.

Counting time beyond a 90 day streak *(privately)* is a Pig's game designed to blow up any tiny mistake into a full-fledged Food Orgy.

But still, if you're not going to rely on counting time as evidence of your ability to abstain forever, how will you deal with insecurity?

After all, your Food Plan is sacred, so you must take any insecurity about complying with it as seriously as you would any impulse to disobey the law. Therefore, if you find the Pig is making you insecure about your ability to stick to your Plan *forever*, make it a priority to identify the Squeal and restore your confidence 100%.

THE ONLY CAUSES OF BINGE ANXIETY

1) **Pig Squeal misidentified as your own thoughts.** To check for this ask yourself: "What _might_ the Pig be trying to get me to believe so I will Binge? What's it saying?" Be specific! Just articulate the Squeal to inoculate yourself in the future. Put it in a Squeal Journal if it helps. Pig Squeal _always_ loses its power in the light of day.

2) **Grey areas your Pig has snuck into your Food Plan.** If you find this is the case, evaluate the Food Plan as per the detailed instructions in the previous chapter.

Binge Anxiety is actually just your Pig's plan to Binge in disguise. Cage the Pig and keep it there!

The question is, do you feel 100%, completely and totally secure in your Food Plan. More importantly, are you 100% confident in your ability to comply with it forever? If not, you either have to find-and-ignore the Pig Squeal or carefully change the Food Plan *(see previous chapter.)* There are NO other options!

It's also important to note, however, that many people wait to get started until they can honestly say they FEEL 100% confident in their plans. These people are confusing their Pig's feelings for their own.

You don't have to FEEL 100% confident. You only have to intellectually believe your Food Plan represents your best thinking at a time when you were of sound mind and were motivated enough to put it all in black and white. Then you DECLARE yourself 100% confident and DECLARE all other thoughts and feelings as belonging to the Pig so you can reject them. And you just take the leap!

This is what I mean when I say Never Binge Again is a "trick of mind." It's just a way of thinking which makes the line between your thin-thinking-self and your fat-thinking alter-ego crystal clear so you can hear the Squeals.

It's a game we play to avoid distracting ourselves with ANY possibility of failure so we can concentrate 100% of our energy on achieving the goal.

Now, to *really* lock down your ability to deal with doubt and insecurity, I'd like to give you a new perspective on deprivation. See, most people's Pigs suggest they won't be able to deal with the feelings of deprivation forever. But there's a LOT more to this notion than appears on the surface...

CHAPTER 7

Overcoming the Deprivation Trap

"You simply can't Never Binge Again. You'll feel way too deprived and eventually you'll just give up and feed me. Why wait? Let's Binge!!!" – Sincerely, Your Pig

"There there now. You're very upset. Go get us some comfort food and let's have ourselves a little Binge. We'll feel SOOOOO much better!" – Sincerely, Your Pig

There are actually TWO types of deprivation: (1) What you deprive yourself of by NOT having something and; (2) what you deprive yourself of by having it. *(To my knowledge, this was first pointed out by Geneen Roth)*

It's exceptionally rare for people to consciously choose between these two alternatives. In fact, most people never consider the second kind at all.

Just for illustration—*I'm NOT saying you have to adopt this rule!*—let's take the notion of never eating donuts again. If you decide to never eat donuts again, you'll deprive yourself of the taste, texture, and mouth feel of a donut for the rest of your natural life. You will never experience donut-pleasure again. To a donut-loving Pig, this is most certainly a fate worse than death.

But if you decide to *continue* eating donuts, you will deprive yourself of everything associated with *never* eating donuts again including (a) acquiring the body of your dreams *(or something very close);* (b) the "lightness of being" associated with life without all that extra weight; (c) the energy associated with more regular, healthy nourishment; (d) knowing what it's like to have consistent blood sugar levels and to live without sugar crashes; (e) the *confidence* which comes from knowing you have the power to NEVER eat a donut again; (f) years near the end of your life which were meant to be pain-free and full of joy, but are instead filled with immobility and dysfunction due to strokes, heart attacks, etc.

Your Pig would love to have you concentrate only on the *short term* effects of deprivation because it genuinely believes Pig Slop is the *only* pleasure life has to offer. But the list of things we deprive ourselves of by *continuing* a food behavior is often a lot longer, and much more painful!

To take advantage of this insight you only need to make a solid comparison between your two choices. What will you deprive yourself of if you continue to embrace the particular food *(or behavior)* vs. assigning it to your Pig's trough?

And I'll tell you what, let's give your Pig a running start by letting it go first. Think about some treat you *just might* want to consider avoiding from now on. Go ahead and tell the Pig to provide you with a long list of things you'll be depriving yourself of if you never eat it again.

Can you feel your Pig squirming? That's because there are only two things it can really put forward in this situation—taste and convenience. Oh, it will say you'll be depriving yourself of life itself—*that you'll starve to death in a matter of hours without its favorite Slop.*

But by now your Pig knows you're on to *that* game. So the best it can do is say "because it tastes good" or "it's so easy to just grab it and go."

Your Pig squirms at the mere thought of this exercise because it knows its ammunition pales in comparison to your side of the equation.

Cage the Pig...write down your list!

Let the Pig say as much as it wants about how deprived you'll feel when you move its Slop to the Nevers section of your Food Plan...

When you write these things down it should become clear to you the Pig is talking about itself. It will feel deprived, not you.

Then write down everything you can think of which YOU will be deprived of by keeping the Pig's Slop in your Plan.

A well-considered, informed decision between the two types of deprivation always favors you, no matter the specifics of the Food Rule under consideration...so just write down the facts and make your choices.

I remember the day I first realized what I was depriving myself of by continuing to eat Pig Slop in a particular situation. I'm kind of an outdoorsman. I haven't won any awards, but for the past 12 years I've driven up to the White Mountain National Forest *(in New Hampshire)* several times a month for a long hike.

Now, a big part of what my Pig used to love about hiking was how much I could feed it without gaining weight. One of my favorite things to do was to hike a 5,000+ foot mountain with a pack full of junk food. And I'd really go to town on my feed bag before, during, and after the hike...

See, my Pig had me convinced there was NO reason to hike without a big sack of Pig Slop. It was as essential as my map, compass, headlamp, and other survival gear...

Then one day, after reading about the two types of deprivation, I realized I literally didn't know what it was like to hike *without* junk food. I hadn't done it even one single day. And I began wondering what I might be missing. So instead of the traditional bags and boxes and bars of crap, I packed up some organic greens and blueberries, put some green tea in a thermos, and threw a bag of raw seeds in my pack.

Here's what happened: An incredible calmness I didn't know anyone could ever feel came over me. As I walked through the woods I felt I could really breathe the air, listen to the running water, appreciate the sites, and enjoy all the animals I encountered. It was one of the best days of my life. It gave me a feeling of "rightness" with the world which since then has been a more powerful lure than anything the Pig can throw at me.

It lasted several days.

I slept better. Felt less reactive to "emergencies" at work. Was better with my clients. Solved problems more easily.

In many ways I felt more present than I'd ever been.

And through this experience I realized it was my Pig who'd convinced me I needed junk food on every hike. But that was a big hairy Pig lie! I'd actually been depriving myself of who I was meant to be at my core.

Since then I've learned this experience of *contentment* is just under the surface for anyone who really wants it. Sadly, most people let their Pigs keep it from them entirely. This upsets me to no end. Why would anyone *ever* choose to Binge when they could just Cage the Pig and keep it there!?

My Pig wanted me to think hiking without Pig Slop was cruel and torturous deprivation. But it turns out I'd been so distracted by the delicious tastes, I had no idea how I truly *was* depriving myself.

Now, if you walk away from this thinking I'm telling you to go hug some trees and avoid any particular food forever, you're missing the point. The point is there are TWO types of deprivation, and you are 100% free to choose either one in any circumstance.

YOU get to choose, not your Pig.

When the Pig says "you can't follow these Food Rules any longer, they're too depriving", pause to ask yourself what the Pig is really aiming to deprive *you* of if you break them.

One last important point about all this...

You make the rules. So be sure you've created a Food Plan you're confident you can live with forever. One which allows you to pursue your dreams in the body you want, while striking the optimal balance between short term pleasures vs. longer term goals. Every rule you make is a compromise between these two ends. Only you can decide where the best line is for your own body—that's what freedom is about!

Here's another way to look at it: Every day we make choices between "Live Fast and Die Young[2]" vs. "Live Slow and Enjoy the Long Ride." Do you want to borrow life from tomorrow to live faster today, or forgo some short term pleasure to achieve a better long term outcome?

In a free country, we have every right to trade suffering *tomorrow* for pleasure *today* if this is what we truly desire. In fact, we've fought wars for this kind of freedom.

However, the problem is most people have allowed their Pigs to dominate these decisions, so they never make a conscious choice. And because they've never experienced long periods of Pig-free eating, they also haven't had the opportunity to make *informed* decisions about these very critical food matters.

I might not agree, but I'd vehemently defend your right to say "I'm choosing to live a little faster right now for the sheer pleasure of it. I'm fully aware I'm probably going to die a little younger and/or suffer more at the end of my life because of this choice, but

---

[2]   This philosophy was first quoted in the 1949 movie "Knock on Any Door" by actor John Derek. The full quote was "Live fast, die young, and leave a good looking corpse"

I'm of sound mind, adult years, and 100% capable of making this conscious choice."

The problem is, people making this tradeoff rarely do so consciously. Instead, they allow their Pigs and society as a whole to pull the wool over their eyes and keep them blind to these choices.

The ultimate responsibility of freedom is choosing whether to live fast and die young vs. enjoy the longer, slower ride. However you decide on any particular Food Rule, please be sure you've given yourself a chance to experience the slower side of the equation so you're making a truly informed choice.

Why? Because the Pig must stay Caged, that's why!

DEPRIVATION WORKSHEET

If you'd like to see exactly what your Pig has been depriving you of and really cement in your defense against the Deprivation Squeal, please download the FREE "Avoiding the Deprivation Trap" workbook at www.NeverBingeAgain.com

CHAPTER 8

Defeating the Food Industry

One day about 15 years ago I was talking with my friend Ted[3]—*successful senior executive in a meal replacement bar company*—about some of his biggest marketing insights. The answer was revealing: One of their most significant growth spurts began when the company REMOVED the vitamins so the bars would taste better, while they simultaneously made the packaging LOOK more nutritious and delicious.

Apparently, it's quite profitable to distract people into THINKING they're eating healthy.

Packaging is only one part of this trend. Another trick of the trade is to emphasize ONE ingredient with proven health benefits in order to distract you from the other harmful ones.

For example, I'm guessing most of you already know fat free foods can still be loaded with sugar. But did you know many "Heart Healthy Omega 3" packaged foods can still have very high levels of sodium? That although dry-roasted nuts may have fewer calories and be lower in unhealthy fats than nuts roasted in oil and sugar—the roasting process itself can still create cancer causing

---

[3]   The real name of my friend and the details of his company have been disguised to protect the innocent.

compounds in significant amounts? That "Whole Grain" labeled products can still be refined enough to spike your blood sugar and increase your risk of diabetes? *(And possibly even cancer?)*

These are just some of the perfectly legal ways the food industry bolsters your Pig's best ideas. It's a "confuse and conquer" strategy. Hundreds of intelligent, high-paid marketing executives, lawyers, consultants, and food scientists are hard at work giving your Pig more ammunition[4]. And why wouldn't they be? To them, your Pig is worth trillions!

Thankfully, all the Food Industry tricks are transparent and easily defeated once you shift your perspective in the simple way I'll share in a moment. And as long as you don't fool yourself, it's perfectly OK to trade a little health for taste, convenience, and enjoyment if that's what YOU really want to do. As long as these are conscious choices made with your fully informed consent, it won't impact your ability to Never Binge Again.

But I need to tread carefully here because most people prefer to arrive at their own conclusions about what constitutes healthy food. And provided the conclusions you arrive at empower you to draw your own unambiguous line in the sand, you can and will make yourself immune to the food industry's tricks. We needn't agree on what constitutes healthy food... you only need to be 100% clear on it for yourself.

Your Pig may chime in here and say:

> "Hey, wait just a minute here Bubba! Glenn said you could create your OWN Food Plan. He said it was entirely up to you... but now he is going to drone on about what's healthy food vs. what's junk. Not only is he lying... but who made *him* the king of health information? See? What have I been telling you! This is all just a bunch of prairie poo. Why are you wasting your time reading it at all? For

---

4   I should know since, sadly, I used to be one of them! My companies have earned tens of millions of dollars consulting for Fortune 500 firms.

God's sake, let's just go Binge already, OK? Can we, can we, can we, can we....please!!!!????"

YOUR FOOD PLAN IS ENTIRELY UP TO YOU –I AM ONLY PROVIDING A SHORTCUT WHICH MIGHT SAVE YOU YEARS OF PAINFUL EXPERIMENTATION. SKIP THE REST OF THIS CHAPTER IF YOU THINK SEEING IT WILL INTERFERE WITH YOUR ABILITY TO INDEPENDENTLY DEFINE HEALTHY FOOD FOR YOURSELF:

THE SIMPLEST WAY TO THINK ABOUT HEALTHY FOOD
(Skip the rest of this chapter if you prefer to come to your own conclusions)

Whole, unprocessed, organic foods are the only genuinely healthy nourishment for humans. Everything else is a man-made refinement for taste, convenience, or enjoyment. Everything. The more refined, better tasting, and convenient a given food is, the more you're likely to be trading on your health for these benefits.

It's much easier to start with a small list of what's good for you *(an affirmative list)* than to make an exhaustive list of what's harmful *(a punitive list of taboos.)* The latter is much too long, complex, and provides the Pig way too much material to debate.

But none of this means you've got to be a saint and just eat dirt and rocks the rest of your life. It's perfectly fine for YOU—not your Pig!—to include choices for taste, convenience, and fun in your Food Plan, with full knowledge you're trading off some health when you do.

Just don't let your Pig fool you into believing the toxic-pleasure peddled by the Food Industry is actually healthy, because that is a recipe for disaster. Whatever you do, resolve right now to deprive your Pig of the constant barrage of well-funded Squeals provided by the food industry's billions.

There's one last critical fact we'll need in order to prevent the food industry from supporting your Pig. After living for decades in a society set up to feed the Pig at every turn, it's likely your natural hunger mechanisms are out of tune with what your body really needs. Your taste buds have been desensitized. The reward pathways in your brain don't fire as intensely in response to the natural foods for which they were designed. They've come to require the more super-rewarding stimulation of processed foods and other societally promoted junk.

But thankfully most of this is reversible. If you eat less sugar, fruit will begin to taste better. As you consume less junk—*as crazy as it sounds!*—you'll begin to find yourself craving green vegetables. But you do NOT have to force these things to happen... and you shouldn't try. They're just a natural result of Never Bingeing Again. Just like someone who quits smoking begins to enjoy deep breaths of clean air like never before, so too will your natural food instincts begin to be revitalized.

The essence of a Pig-hijacked survival drive is the belief your Binge food is a fundamental requirement for life itself. To make room for this, the Pig rejects what nature actually has to offer. But when you cage the Pig, this process slowly but surely reverses itself.

One last thing on this point which your Pig will hate: There's overwhelming evidence which suggests raw, organic, leafy greens are to nutrition what oxygen is to your lungs. So if you want to speed up the recovery and re-normalization of your survival drive, just add some to your diet. You can throw them in the blender with a little water and drink them down like medicine. You don't have to enjoy them, you just need to get them in. When you add organic leafy greens, you begin to crowd out everything else.

But if you find this suggestion too aversive, please know it's not a requirement and there's NO need to force it. No matter what your Food Plan, if you keep Caging Your Pig you should naturally begin evolving towards healthy food.

The reason I'm so confident about this is because the places you'll naturally choose to cage the Pig are those in which you experience the most unpleasant side effects of toxic pleasure. As you eliminate more and more toxic pleasure from your diet, you'll naturally gravitate towards getting your nutrition from healthier foods. You can't help it any more than a smoker could help breathing in real oxygen after they quit poisoning their lungs with cigarettes.

When a smoker quits smoking, those large, slow, deep breaths of fresh air can make them a lot more comfortable. They can still quit forever regardless of whether they embrace this practice, but life is a lot easier if they do. Similarly, you can dominate the Pig forever without eating your stupid vegetables. But things will go faster and you'll make life easier if you do.

Enough said!

THE FIVE MOST COMMON FOOD INDUSTRY LIES

If you'd really like to bolster your defense against the food industry's Pig-feeding tricks, please download my free audio *(and word for word transcript): "The Five Most Common Food Industry Lies and How to Defeat Them!"* from www.NeverBingeAgain.com

CHAPTER 9

"Hell is Other People[5]"
(Says Your Pig)

In the past few decades psychologists have discovered our self-concept is intimately bound with how others see us. None of us seem to know who we are until we see it reflected in someone else's eyes. As if self-worth can only derive from the mirror of other people's thoughts, feelings, and opinions.

While it may be true we can't avoid having our self-concept *influenced* by our relationships, your Pig takes this to a ludicrous extreme. It wants you to believe the slightest instability in your loved ones' opinions about you and/or your Food Plan will cause you to Binge.

In other words, your new Food Plan will upset your wife, your children, your mom, your husband, your grandma, your second cousin, your nephew, and of course your dog. *(Don't forget your dog!)* And without their 100% unconditional acceptance of everything you do, the Pig says you'll be incapable of sticking to a simple commitment. So you might as well give up and Binge.

---

[5] Hell is Other People" comes from Jean Paul Sartre's existentialist play "No Exit" where the characters are forced to spend eternity in one room fruitlessly seeking themselves in each other.

Pig Squeal!

> ➢ As a side note, it's also entirely possible you could upset your wife, mom, second cousin, *(or dog)* by <u>including</u> something in your Food Plan which they think should never be eaten. In fact, if we were truly dependent on other's opinions to stick to our Food Plan NO food would ever be acceptable—*because if you look hard enough you'll find someone who believes you should never have it.*

Here's the thing: You are perfectly, 100% capable of drawing lines in the sand regardless of what anyone does around you. If you decide you're never going to eat a particular food again, then your wife, mother, father, grandfather and/or dog could bake the most delicious Pig Slop you can imagine and wave it in front of your nose saying "C'mon... just one little bite? It's really, really good. One little bite never killed anyone!"...

And you could still say "no thank you" from here to eternity.

When others tempt you with food, just quietly say *to yourself* "That's Pig Slop...and I Will Never Eat Pig Slop Again!"

It's important to reiterate this is not something you share out loud. Your Food Plan is a very private and personal matter. You don't need to debate, justify, and/or explain it to another soul in the universe.

By extension, other people's Food Plans are also none of your business. Telling someone else they're eating Pig Slop is a great way to ruin a good relationship...

Everyone gets to decide for themselves what goes in their Pig's trough vs. their human plate. In fact, everyone gets to decide whether they want to separate their addictive mind from their more constructive thoughts and feelings in the first place.

We all also get to decide for ourselves whether to call a Pig into existence *at all.* So you've got NO way of knowing whether the person you're talking to wants to even acknowledge their own

Pig...much less to discern how this person defines Pig Slop in their own personal Food Plan.

Only our own Pigs are truly knowable. To mess with other people's Pigs without their permission is an intrusive type of mind-reading.

Besides, having practiced psychology for decades, I can tell you mind-reading is NO easy feat. Just when I think I know what someone's thinking, I manage to hold off and listen a little while longer and discover I was actually way off the mark. Even with people I've known for years.

And even if you COULD see another person's Pig with 100% accuracy, that doesn't make it OK to point out. After all, Superman didn't go around telling everyone he knew what kind of underwear they were wearing even though he had x-ray vision.

So please resist the urge to tell other people they're eating Pig Slop.

If they push back when you say "no thank you" to something and you need more ammunition to make them stop annoying you, you can always say it's for medical reasons. The Food Plan you've adopted will always have something to do with your *physiological* well-being, so you'll always have medical reasons for maintaining it—if for no other reason than a healthy Food Plan is almost certainly medically necessary to maintain a healthy body! *(Even one Binge of most types of Pig Slop can cause sharp spikes in numerous medical risk factors)*

If the other person asks "what medical reasons?" just say "Oh, I'm not dying or anything like that, but I kind of hate talking about it" and then change the topic. That'll usually do it unless your loved one is a real sicko with food. And if they *are* a real sicko, why entertain their ideas in the first place?

People have food trouble with others in their social environment because they unknowingly allow their Pigs to go around seeking approval.

Remember, one of the biggest problems in food addiction is dependency, which provides the perfect excuse for a Binge:

> "So and so seduced you into Bingeing, so you can't possibly blame yourself. It was just too hard to keep to your Food Plan given how much (s)he wanted you to eat _____. Besides, it was really yummy! Let's get more!!!" – How your Pig uses other people as an excuse

The defense against this is to make your Food Plan a 100% private matter. You don't need anyone to validate it.

You might seek education from your doctor, nutritionist, and other experts you respect. And you might read nutritional books to continue amassing information about healthy eating.

But there's NO reason to talk to anyone else about it.

In fact, you should be very careful even talking to experts unless and until you've fully vetted them, and are sure their opinions have not been overly distorted by the profit motive.

In the end, YOU assume full responsibility for your Food Plan, no matter how well informed you are by experts. After all, it's your body.

See, when it comes to eating, other people aren't "Hell", they're just a minor annoyance.

You could stand in a kitchen full of gourmet chefs—*completely surrounded with the most delicious appetizers, entrees, and deserts*—while they all tempt your Pig for hours...*without breaking a single rule on your Food Plan!* Because once you've eliminated ambiguity from your Food Plan then every tempting comment can immediately be recognized as Pig Squeal, and all the "treats" offered become obvious Pig Slop in *your* model of the world.

Therefore, when others are tempting your Pig in a social dining environment just look at the treat and say to yourself "That is Pig Slop. And I Will Never Eat Pig Slop Again!" If the Pig keeps

Squealing then give it the middle finger and coldly say "That's just how it is, Pig!!!"

The more information you have about how to dominate the Pig, the more you're going to realize it's the PIG that's powerless, NOT you!!

What Your Pig Says About Being Influenced by Others Around Food	What YOU Say About Being Influenced by Others Around Food
"Hell is other people! You can't be around other people and stick to your Food Plan because you'll upset them too much. We'll just have to have ourselves a yummy, yummy Binge when we see them and start over the next day."	"The Hell with other people! There isn't one single soul on this planet who can convince me to eat Pig Slop because I will NEVER eat Pig Slop *again... and that's that!*"

Now, before we leave this chapter on dealing with other people, let me just say it IS possible to introduce willing participants to the Never Binge Again philosophy. Here's how you do it...

Wait until you come across someone who's actively concerned about their weight and/or eating behavior. In other words, they're experiencing the immediate, painful after-effects of toxic pleasure — OR — they are significantly impressed with your results.

In this situation, your friend may be amenable to hearing about the **results** you've achieved using a very different and powerful approach. Make sure they know this approach lets you define your own Food Plan and does NOT impose any particular dietary rules.

It's best if you can get them to read the book *(always available at* www.NeverBingeAgain.com*)* before going into too much detail, or their Pig may talk them out of reading it. Thereafter, if they seem intrigued and give you permission, it can be very gratifying to help them identify their Pig's Squeals...

But if they seem to be rejecting the Never Binge Again philosophy there's really not much you can do. In these cases it's best to say "I'm sorry it wasn't helpful" and politely change the topic.

Fighting with other people's Pigs is NOT a winnable war unless you have a clear ally, and the collateral damage is too great when you don't. When in doubt, just have your friend read the book and see what they think.

(Note: There's nothing wrong with telling a spouse or other loved one that their wellbeing impacts you and your family. Sometimes it takes the withdrawal of affection to get people to change. Sometimes they won't change no matter what you do, and you'll need to consider whether the relationship itself has become toxic. But you won't get anywhere by trying to force the Never Binge Again philosophy on them. In fact, doing so can ruin the possibility they'll consider it at a later juncture. "A man convinced against his will is of the same opinion still" – Samuel Butler)

Because the super-rewarding food our society has produced is indeed SUPER delicious, Never Binge Again is experienced as a pretty radical concept which most people will only be open to when they're really in pain. And when they are, it's necessary to get a LOT of information into their heads reasonably quickly with a certain amount of practiced finesse.

For this reason, it's better to leave the education to the book itself *(and/or the audios and videos on the* www.NeverBingeAgain.com *website)* when possible. Dominating your own Pig and teaching others to do the same are two entirely different matters. The ideas in Never Binge Again are NOT very contagious... most people unfortunately need to have been beaten down fairly seriously by their Pigs before they will be open to them.

Let's talk for a few minutes about what's necessary to TEACH someone else to Never Binge Again by reviewing how I got you to accept the idea while reading this book. *(I know, I know, your Pig may still Squeal that you haven't made up your mind yet—stupid Pig. Cage the Pig!)*

First, I carefully sold you on the concept of the Pig during the introduction. I explained how this could work for you where nothing had ever worked before. Then I made an outrageous promise: If you'd be willing to entertain a crazy idea—*with suspended judgment*—I could give you control over your eating *forever*. And I explained you only needed to let me provide you with a weird idea to ponder for a while in order to benefit. It wasn't another grit-your-teeth-and-bear it exhausting diet.

Only with this motivation in place could we proceed to carefully define the Pig, outlining how it was possible to make this seemingly irrational leap without giving up your ability to think clearly[6].

The next step was to forewarn you of the impending violent backlash you might experience against these ideas. Why? Because Pigs Squeal loudly and frantically as soon as they realize we're on to their game. And at that juncture you hadn't yet separated your own thoughts from Pig Squeal—so the Pig could have easily dissuaded you from reading further.

Because the Pig's best-first-line of attack is to destroy the concept before it even takes hold, we had to create a safe channel for the Pig Squeal while we educated you about its tricks. This was the first step in leading your Pig into its forever prison.

And this is perhaps the most difficult part about teaching other people to see their own Pigs: Before deciding to call a Pig into existence, people are in an undifferentiated state. They haven't yet separated from their own fat thinking thoughts. Before understanding the Never Binge Again concept, those thoughts are still an integral part of who they are and what they value as a human being. *Therefore, the idea of separating from this bothersome part of themselves is at first experienced as a very harsh criticism of their own personhood.*

---

[6] In fact, when you do it right, dominating the Pig actually improves your reasoning ability!!

In other words, at the beginning a newbie's Pig's violent struggle for survival is perceived as *their own*. This makes them prone to arguing with you if you present the idea too forcefully. And since the Pig is a SURVIVAL drive run-amuck, the energy behind this argument is the same energy behind the thrashing of a drowning person. It may be politely hidden, but their Pigs will say and/or do ANYTHING to survive.

For all these reasons it's best to get this book into your prospective Pig Dominator's hands rather than undertake the battle yourself.

Notwithstanding the above, people can and will accept the notion of a Pig after they've taken a particularly strong beating by their food struggles. They have to really want results, and feel a little desperate to find a different solution[7].

For all these reasons, for many people the Pig is a concept which just gets planted and grows over time. Be prepared for push back. And just like it's fruitless to argue and debate with your own Pig, don't become too argumentative with theirs. Let the book do the hard work...then let them have their say thereafter.

Some people will love you for this! And it's *very* exciting to be around others who have truly committed to Never Binge Again.

But it's important to remember these people will probably define their own Food Plans very much differently than you defined yours. What sounds like Pig Squeal to you may indeed be healthy thinking for them. And what looks like Pig Slop to you may be perfectly good food in their view of the world. That's fine – you're separate and unique individuals with separate and unique Food Plans!

Others will want to push aside the concept and continue struggling as they have been, looking for that magic formula which allows

---

7   Note: They do NOT have to "hit bottom"...but they do have to have sufficient motivation. *(Waiting to "hit bottom" is a type of Pig Squeal in and of itself. The Pig says "I guess you haven't hit bottom yet. Let's just keep Bingeing until you do. Yummy!!!")*

them to have their cake and eat it too. It's OK. Let them. You've planted a seed which they may remember the next time they're stung by toxic pleasure.

Regardless of what other people in your life do, just Never Binge Again!

UNUSUAL WAYS TO NEUTRALIZE OTHER PEOPLE'S PIGS

If you'd like to supercharge your defense against other people's Pigs, download my free audio *(and transcript)* "Unusual Ways to Neutralize Other People's Pigs" from www.NeverBingeAgain.com

CHAPTER 10

The Pig is Powerless, Not You

A good portion of our society believes there's a mysterious disease which makes certain people completely powerless over food, alcohol, drugs, and other toxic pleasures. Spokespeople from the addiction treatment industry often suggest that super-rewarding foods trigger an irresistible impulse which "compulsive overeaters" are powerless to defend themselves against.

If you're one of these diseased people, as this line of reasoning goes, you can't ever hope to control yourself, and you certainly can't quit eating any particular food. The best you can hope for is "one day at a time" abstinence while you dedicate the rest of your life to hanging around with others *(who also can't control themselves)* so you can all supposedly watch over one another...

And help each other through the inevitable string of "relapses" to come, since you are, after all, just a slave to your disease, doomed to a lifetime of Bingeing and recovery. *(An institutionalized rationale to remove responsibility and guilt, claim ongoing helplessness, and taking a permanent position as a victim)*

"What a delicious disease!!!"
(Says Your Pig)

There's NO good scientific, empirical evidence for this mysterious disease.

The disease concept was originally put forth by Alcoholics Anonymous to reduce guilt and shame over indulgences which put the lives, finances, and wellbeing of not only the drinker but also their family at risk. It was easier for families to accept their loved one was suffering from a disease than to think of them as an arrogant and selfish person who risked life, limb, and the security of the family for just one more drinking binge.

The idea of powerlessness has now been extended to virtually every imaginable toxic pleasure. People say—*and our culture willingly accepts*—there are diseases which make some of us powerless over alcohol, drugs, gambling, infidelity, sexual perversions, and pretty much anything else that feels good[8].

Of course, this extends to food.

"It's not our fault and it's not a moral issue" says the current chorus of voices from the addiction treatment industry. "And relapse is an inevitable part of recovery"

Poppycock.

Here's the thing: Human beings are perfectly capable of abstaining from toxic pleasure. **Pigs are powerless over people, NOT the other way around.** And the most glaring evidence of this is that the Pig bothers to talk at all.

We already know the Pig wants only to Binge, and will SAY whatever it takes to convince you to feed it. But did you ever stop to think why it bothers with all the verbal mumbo jumbo in the first place? If all it wants is Pig Slop, why not just quietly go and take some? Why must it say anything at all?

---

[8] Can you have a "red light running disease", for example? Could you be a compulsive bowler?

Because the Pig CAN'T feed itself, that's why! It's a powerless creature whose only hope is to get you to go along with its warped thinking. That's why it's always desperately trying to convince you to get its junk. That's why it talks a blue streak until it realizes you will Never Binge Again.

THE VERY FACT THE PIG TALKS PROVES YOU ARE ITS JAILOR. IT'S COMPLETELY POWERLESS TO FEED ITSELF, SO IT'S ONLY HOPE FOR RELEASE IS VERBALLY CONVINCING YOU TO LET IT OUT OF PRISON.

Here's something very nice to know: Even—*and perhaps especially*—if the Pig should ever happen to be correct about any particular point, you will still NEVER Binge again. You will NEVER grant it control over your arms, legs, or mouth.

Because regardless of what it says, the Pig only wants to indulge in toxic pleasures which will destroy everything you care about. So who cares if the Pig went out and got a degree from Harvard—or for that matter, if it found the cure for cancer? You'd still ignore every last Squeal because you know it has only this one destructive motive.

The Pig is a weak, single-minded creature which doesn't care about anything besides Bingeing. It will extract any price from your life to get at its Slop, but it's completely powerless to do so unless you listen to its Squeals.

The Pig is powerless and you are its master.

So turn a deaf ear and just Never Binge Again!

(Note: I'm legally required to inform you that notwithstanding what's said in this chapter there are some serious eating disorders— including but not limited to bulimia and anorexia—which do require professional assistance. Only a licensed professional can diagnose these disorders and prescribe the appropriate treatment)

CHAPTER 11

Hard to Recognize Pig Squeals!

O nce you've begun to dominate the Pig, it will begin watching for an opportunity to break out of its cage. That's its job! So in this chapter we'll review some fairly common—*but hard to recognize*—Pig Squeals which many people have trouble hearing at first.

Like all Squeals, these twelve fall apart when examined in the light of day. Nevertheless, arming yourself with foreknowledge of the most common Pig Costumes used shortly after resolving to Never Binge Again can be very helpful.

And although I'll take the time to disprove each of them, please remember this is overkill and simply for the point of illustration— *kind of like slicing a watermelon with a chainsaw when a simple knife would do...*

You do NOT need to memorize, recall and present these perfect arguments to your Pig because your mind is not a debate club or a democracy. It's a monarchy, and you are the King *(or Queen.)* The Pig is nothing more than your obedient peasant. It must comply with your every rule no matter how silly or unnecessary it may seem.

You make the laws. The Pig has no choice but to obey.

For this reason, simply acknowledging Pig Squeal as Pig Squeal is more than sufficient to inoculate you against this peasant, your majesty...

But you do need to recognize them first. So let's start with the trickiest Squeal of all.

THE HARDEST SQUEAL TO RECOGNIZE

One of the early changes most people observe when they decide to cage the Pig is a remarkably improved ability to get back on track faster if they happen to make a mistake. What most people don't expect, however, is that the Pig will attempt to hijack this ability for its own purpose. As soon as the Pig realizes you're feeling more confident about getting back on track after a Binge it will say something like:

> "Hey! You're getting really good at putting me back in my cage using this new dominate the Pig stuff, so I really can't do too much harm anymore. After all, you can just lock me back up whenever you feel like it. So how about let's go have ourselves a great big hairy Bingeing party, you and me, OK? That's what we've been wanting all these years anyway, isn't it? Finally! A safe way to Binge! Thank God for Never Binge Again because now we can do it!!!" –Your Pig

Listen, your word is sacred.

A Binge is ALWAYS a big deal.

You made a solemn oath to follow a Food Plan. It doesn't matter how small a transgression your Pig has in mind. Your word is your word. Period.

If you give the Pig an inch it will try to take a mile and you know it. Let it land on the beach and it will marshal all its troops to fortify its position and take as much of your territory as possible. The Pig will always do its best to turn "just one bite" into a week-long Food Orgy.

Which is why NEVER means NEVER.

Cage the Pig!!

HARD TO RECOGNIZE SQUEAL #2

"90% compliance is good enough. After all, you used to eat badly a LOT more often. Why not leave well-enough alone?" – Your Pig

Giving the Pig 10% leeway only creates the opportunity for it to take more, and more, and more. And I can prove it:

- ➢ 90% today times 90% tomorrow brings you to 81% of your original goal. *(90% x 90% = 81%)*

- ➢ The next day you're down to 72.9% *(81% x 90% = 72.9%)*

- ➢ By the end of the week you'll be at LESS THAN HALF of your original plan. *(90% x 90% x 90% x 90% x 90% x 90% x 90% = 47.8%)*

- ➢ Follow this logic to its natural conclusion and in just one month you'll be at a miserable 4.2%

If you comply 90%, you'll be back in Full Binge Mode within thirty days!

90% is Pig Squeal, plain and simple.

100% is the ONLY possible solution.

Anything less than a 100% commitment is nothing more than the Pig's plan to Binge.

- ➢ You don't set out to climb a mountain saying "maybe I will and maybe I won't." You visualize yourself on top and you commit.

- ➢ You don't get married saying "maybe this will work and maybe it won't." Either you feel strongly enough to commit 100% or you find yourself a different mate.

> ➤ You don't get in a car saying "maybe I'll get to my destination safely or maybe I'll crash." You commit 100% to avoiding other vehicles *(and anything else not-so-good-for-humans-in-cars.)*

> ➤ You don't drink clean water 90% of the time, but have yourself a big old swig from the toilet the other 10%.

A 90% committed athlete will almost never make it out of the minor leagues. To have any chance of taking home the gold you've got to give it your all.

Now let's talk about 100%.

100% commitment doesn't degrade over time. If you commit 100% today, you'll still be at 100% tomorrow because 100% x 100% still equals 100%. And you know what? You'll be at 100% the next day too. *(100% x 100% x 100% = 100%)*. Ad infinitum.

Commit 100% each and every day and you'll be at 100% on the very last day of your life because 100% to the power of infinity is still 100%.

100% is the ONLY number which does this.

Even 99% eventually degrades to full Binge mode...it just takes a little longer. *(You'd be at less than half your plan in under three-months-time, and down to almost zero by the end of the year)*

Moreover, the slight edge you get from a 100% vs. 90% commitment may not seem like much the first few days, but it compounds over time.

A 100% committed athlete rises to the top of their game even though they may only edge out their competition by a nose on any particular day. Their slight edge day after day after day adds up. Because winning by just a nose every time is still winning, they *really* stand out from the crowd. It's not unusual for such athletes to get ten times more recognition and compensation than their peers.

The slight edge in confidence YOU will get from complying 100% makes all the difference in your Pig understanding it will NEVER win vs. thinking it will only be a matter of time. And when the Pig knows it will NEVER win, it will eventually conclude it has no choice but to give up and leave you alone.

But at 90% compliance the Pig keeps Squealing. It drains your energy and confidence and wears you down. 90% always leads to a low self-esteem Binge mentality over time. At 90% the Pig never knows when it's going to hit that "lucky 10%." So it acts like a frantic gambler glued to a slot machine in Vegas, dedicating ALL its energy just to be sure it's still in the game to pull the lever when that "one big win" comes due.

Even at 99.9999% compliance the Pig will, in fact, continue this behavior. Because one chance in a million—*or a billion for that matter!*—is enough to give the Pig hope. And a little hope is all the Pig needs to keep going.

Think of how many tens of millions of people buy lottery tickets each week because "Hey, you never know" *(NY lottery slogan)* or "you've got to be in it to win it!"

But just as a prisoner serving a life sentence eventually decides hope is undesirable and painful, at 100% compliance your Pig will eventually let go of hope so you get on with your life.

And it happens a lot sooner than you might think!

Therefore, it's in your best interest to quash every last ray of hope your Pig may be holding onto in order to live a confident, Binge-free life...*forevermore.*

When you accept 90% compliance, you're depriving yourself of the immense confidence and peace of mind which only 100% can bring.

100% is really the ONLY option.

You must be willing to pay ANY price to achieve 100% compliance with your own Food Plan... and your Pig must know this with certainty.

Remember, it's YOU who wrote the Food Plan in the first place! What's the point of not 100% complying with yourself? Isn't the whole point of freedom being able to chart ANY course you want and successfully reach the destination?

In this context, I hope you can see how STUPID the Pig is for incessantly trying to talk you out of this.

HARD TO RECOGNIZE SQUEAL #3

"The sheer number of times you've previously Binged despite your most sacred promises and commitments— *even after reading this book*—proves you'll never be able to stick to ANY Food Plan whatsoever. You're just too weak. Face it, you've already tried to dominate me and failed. How many more times are you going to do this before you accept it's impossible? Just give up and accept a life of Bingeing until our hearts are content. Yummmmmmm!!!!" – Your Pig

Even if you've repeatedly fallen down for years, continuing to get up until you succeed is a mark of strength, not weakness!

A weak person gives in and gives up, but people who chose to keep renewing their vow to *forever* lock the Pig in its cage until that lock becomes unbreakable can't help but succeed. Renewed commitment is a mark of fortitude and perseverance. It's something to be revered, not ridiculed!

The fact you've fought a biological error your whole life and experimented with dozens of ideas for a Food Plan before making your FINAL one is admirable...

And as long as you're 100% committed to utterly and completely dominating the Pig, you will continue to make steady progress until you beat it into permanent submission.

In fact, this occurred just after your *last* Binge, no matter whether that was 5 seconds, 5 minutes, or 5 years ago!

The Pig would like to use your past mistakes as evidence of permanent weakness—*and it will most certainly jump on the chance to attack any mistakes you may make after reading this book*—but in doing so it actually draws attention to your fortitude and persistence.

The Pig makes your point *for* you.

Stupid Pig!

You are 100% capable of making an irreversible decision, regardless of how many times you may have reversed the same decision before. This is true even if, as a practical matter, some people require a multitude of attempts before arriving at their FINAL Food Plan.

HARD TO RECOGNIZE SQUEAL #4
(The "Controlled Bingeing" Strategy)

> The Pig says: "A planned and controlled Binge once in a while isn't so bad. That's what you intend to do anyway and you know it. You can Binge one out of ten meals and still get thin. So what's the problem? Let's go already, I'm ready when you are. And it'll be SO yummy!!!"
> –Your Pig

A Binge is defined as even one bite or swallow outside of your carefully constructed Food Plan. Nobody told you what to put on this Plan. It represents your best thinking at a time when you were of sound mind and felt motivated enough to write it down. With great forethought, you defined a set of clear rules you firmly believed were in your best interest.

REMEMBER: There's nothing which says you can't have good tasting, delicious foods <u>on</u> your Plan. It's even perfectly legitimate to include things you know are unhealthy if YOU want to make those trade-offs...

But it's *your* plan, not the Pig's!

Which is why it's imperative you recognize this particular Squeal as the Pig's attempt to intrude on your best thinking. The Pig hates your well-considered ideas because the only way it will ever get fed is if it can get you to act on impulse. But...

There's absolutely NO need for "Cheat Days" and/or "Controlled Binges" on a well-considered Food Plan which nobody forced you to adopt in the first place. *(You CAN have "Special Days" where you conditionally allow a loosening of your regular rules in a pre-thought out and well articulated manner. For example "I Only Ever Eat Chocolate on Sundays." But "Cheating" implies breaking the rules and that's NOT something we want your Pig to think is EVER a possibility!)*

You've already used your own best thinking to create a balanced plan for health, well-being, and enjoyment. If you're unhappy with it, go back and change it according to the procedure we've already discussed. But the sudden idea to have a controlled departure is nothing more than a plan to Binge. And you know where *that* slovenly idea is coming from, don't you!?

Remember: If you plan it in as part of your Food Rules then it's NOT Pig Slop in the first place.

You Will Never Eat Pig Slop Again!

You Will Never Binge Again!

HARD TO RECOGNIZE SQUEAL #5
("I Don't Really Exist")

> "You know there's not really a Pig inside you. Therefore none of this 'Dominate the Pig' stuff makes ANY sense at all. So why don't you just let me out and Binge already!!!?"
> – Your Pig

As discussed previously, the Pig is a language gimmick. There's no *real* Pig inside you. It's only a concept, even though the dynamic between you and the Pig can be characterized as that which exists between more recently evolved neocortical functions and the mid-brain, where survival impulses originate.

But the Pig is not "just" a language gimmick, it's an *incredibly effective* language gimmick! In fact, it may be the ONLY way to thoroughly separate your thin-thinking-self from the fat thoughts and feelings which have sabotaged your efforts until this point in life.

And let's bring back our governmental analogy: The continually refined use of language is what allows humans to coordinate and control their impulses so they can participate in a civil society. Language is what separates us from the apes and allows us to articulate the laws which make it possible to live amongst one another.

Language is how we managed to step out of the jungle and move beyond "might makes right" to form a society.

Language is the very fabric of our civilization.

Never Binge Again is a way of using language which can restore full control over your eating, and eradicate the ridiculous notion that free will and responsibility don't exist when it comes to toxic pleasure.

The Pig would love you to declare it non-existent so it could Binge.

Cage the Pig and keep it there!

HARD TO RECOGNIZE SQUEAL #6
(The "We Can Only Be Grateful Squeal")

"Wanting and striving are useless. Learning to love what you have is the only thing which leads to happiness. Besides, there's ONE super-duper-wonderful thing we can always be grateful for...Pig Slop! Yummy!!!!! Gimmeee some!!!!" – Your Pig

This Squeal is hard to recognize because it actually contains a significant half-truth: Being grateful for what you have IS an important part of a content and satisfied life. It starkly contrasts with harboring resentments, envy, and jealously for others' accomplishments and possessions.

That said, without striving and yearning nobody would ever accomplish *anything*. Feeling uncomfortable about the gap between where we are and where we want to be is what causes people to set goals and make plans in the first place.

A healthy person actively tolerates a certain amount of discomfort and uses it as motivation to change. They set clear goals and diligently work towards them over time. A well person admires the characteristics of others who've achieved and obtained things they themselves desire—*and tries to adopt these characteristics so they might achieve similarly.*

Yes, a well person IS grateful for what they have along the way, but they don't allow this gratefulness to interfere with their striving.

There are three ways people deviate from the well attitude described above... and each of them supports the Pig in its efforts:

> ➢ DEVIATION #1 – ENVY AND RAGE: Some people become driven by rage and envy in the face of other people's accomplishments. They harbor tremendous resentment and believe others aren't entitled to the success they've achieved. It's "unfair", they reason. "Those" people are just lucky, and they themselves can't ever catch a break. And they're not going to take this lying down, either! The envious, enraged person feels justified in attempting to destroy the accomplishments of others, or at least in preventing them from feeling good about what they've done. They want to steal the spoils of the accomplished person's efforts—or prevent them from accomplishing anything in the first place. Such people dedicate themselves to *getting even* instead of being well. And this position fuels

the Pig's argument that the only thing worth living for is Pig Slop.

> DEVIATION #2 – NEGATIVITY AND DEPRESSION: Other people become self-castigating. They wallow in negativity, depression, and self-criticism. The Pig then uses this as justification for indulging in Pig Slop as the *only* good thing in life.

> DEIVATION #3 – EXCESSIVE GRATEFULNESS: The third way people can deal with the discomfort of the gap between where they are and where they'd like to be is Over-Gratefulness. It goes something like this:

✓ "Forget your big goals entirely. There's no point planning for anything long term because you never know when we're going to be spending days, weeks, or months in a full-fledged Food Orgy. The best we can ever hope for is to avoid becoming angry, resentful, or negative. Therefore, we should only focus on being grateful for the shadow of a life we can manage to cobble together between Bingeing episodes. Besides, there's always the next yummy Binge to look forward to, right? Right!!!" – Your Pig

NONE of these three deviations are a smart idea.

It's all well and good to be grateful and shun negativity, but the Pig would have you focus on this exclusively. If it succeeds, it will remove your motivation to pursue longer terms goals with the diligence and discipline it takes to achieve them. And since you won't be accomplishing much to speak of using this Piggy philosophy of life, Pig Slop will start to seem like a good idea.

The Pig hates when you diligently plan and persevere towards your goals because it knows accomplishing them will make Pig Slop—*and all the suffering associated with it*—progressively less attractive as time goes on.

Knowing You Will NEVER Binge Again, on the other hand, allows you to make plans and pursue dreams you couldn't even imagine while you were letting your Pig run the show.

> ➢ Aiming High + Planning + Diligence + Persistence + Gratefulness = Happy Life.

> ➢ Gratefulness Only = Opening the Pig's Cage

Keep the Pig in its Cage!

HARD TO RECOGNIZE SQUEAL #7

"You just Binged. Shame on you! Now you must suffer with constant obsession and excessive guilt about all the bad foods you ate and what a bad person you are. *(At least we'll get to keep thinking about those delicious foods. And besides, once you've done enough penance you'll have paid the price and we'll be clear to Binge again. I can't wait!!!!)*" - Sincerely, Your Pig

It's only natural to feel a degradation in self-esteem and confidence when you've broken your solemn word to yourself or others. But normal, healthy guilt is only supposed to bring your attention to an area which needs improvement. Once you understand and commit to what needs to be improved—*for example if you've identified the specific Pig Attack and have recommitted to your Food Plan*—then guilt has served its function and it's time to move on.

A well person feels guilt and shame when they let themselves or others down. They see it as a signal to examine their behavior and find significant ways to improve. But thereafter holding onto guilt is a Pig's game. *Excessive* guilt is a type of penance the Pig wants you to focus on so you can "pay the price" for the *next* Binge.

In your world there's NO price worth paying for a Binge. But the Pig thinks even one tiny bite or swallow of Pig Slop is worth ANY price. So it muddies the issue. What the Pig is really saying in this particular Squeal is:

"Go ahead and beat yourself up while you keep thinking about all the delicious junk we ate. If that's the price we have to pay to get some Pig Slop again, so be it!" – Your Pig

REMEMBER: To Never Binge Again all you need to do is Never Binge Again. You do not need to repeatedly smack yourself in the head with a spatula to prove you've suffered enough.

"Hey, there's an idea! Why don't we punish ourselves doubly hard for this last Binge? That way we'll have enough punishment stored up to get away with one more...FREE! Good thinking there Bubba![9]" – *How your Pig motivates you to keep punishing yourself for a Binge*

You don't need to write a novel about your Binge. You don't need to go confess in the town square.

Yes, you allowed the Pig to misdirect your energy and harm your body with some Pig Slop. But after you've identified the Pig Attack *(or problem in your Food Plan)* it's a complete waste of time to dwell on guilt and shame about the Binge because you will NEVER Binge again and that's that.

Your body will recover within a day or two, and along with it, your confidence.

HARD TO RECOGNIZE SQUEAL #8
("You Can Exercise Off the Calories")

"You'll exercise enough to justify this Binge later on today. Or maybe you already did. Or we could do it tomorrow. Who cares... it's yummy. Let's go!!!" – Sincerely – Your Pig

One of the Pig's most idiotic arguments is that it's perfectly fine to eat Pig Slop because there's enough time left in the day to exercise off the calories. Or perhaps *after* a good exercise session the Pig may suggest you've "earned it." Or maybe you will do

---

[9] My Pig calls me Bubba. I don't really know why.

enough exercise *tomorrow*. Or next year. Or maybe when you're 99 years old. *("Yeah, that's the ticket! Let's Binge until we're 99 and then spend one year making up for it at the end of our lives. That sounds like a plan, Stan!" – Your Pig)*

Here's the problem: Anything even .00001% off your Food Plan poisons everything important to you. There are always physical effects beyond calories and weight loss...such as fatigue, difficulty working the next day, and the need to eat more over and above the cheat to rebalance your blood sugar, sodium levels, etc.

Pig Slop is Pig Slop and a Binge is a Binge. It doesn't matter how much exercise you've done today, will do tomorrow, or plan to do sometime in the next 99 years. You will avoid Pig Slop from here to eternity as if it were poison. You'd never consciously consume some arsenic with the idea you could exercise it off later, so why do it with Slop?

HARD TO RECOGNIZE SQUEAL #9

"You really must eat something off your plan
every once in a while or you'll starve!"
Sincerely – Your Pig

If you never eat Pig Slop again—*and you never will*—the PIG will starve and YOU will thrive! Cage the Pig!

HARD TO RECOGNIZE SQUEAL #10

"I'm not an idiot. I'm just as smart as you are. And, OK, I'll admit it... I DO exist inside you after all. So you really need to listen to my incredibly intelligent, complex arguments for Bingeing because I'm just as likely to be right as you are. Besides, you really *want* to hear me out so we can Binge, don't you? Let's go!!!" – Your Pig

Because the Pig derives from a survival drive which is indeed anatomically inside of you, it has access to the full force of your native intelligence. But that's NOT a good reason to listen to it!

YOU use intelligence to accomplish worthy goals and aspirations. The Pig uses it for destructive purposes only.

To engage in debate over the merit of the Pig's arguments is like talking to a serial killer about the merit of their deeds. Save your energy for those who have more constructive aims. Nothing good ever comes from letting a serial killer win an argument. Even if he's right!

Even if the Pig is not an idiot, you must treat it as if it were.

The Pig will use ALL the intellectual capacity it can borrow from your brain to argue for indulgence. Its ultimate aim is to obliterate your human ability to delay gratification and thoughtfully direct your behavior—*and instead have you behave like a dog in a meat factory.*

No matter how smart your Pig may appear, it is NOT trying to win an intellectual debate at Harvard. There's only one purpose to its debate: To get you acting like a wild animal...

If you fail to treat the Pig like an idiot it will treat YOU like an idiot!

It's idiotic to give human rights and responsibilities to an animal. We don't give driver's licenses to dogs *(or let them vote.)* We certainly don't give them free access to the refrigerator, the butcher's shop, or the supermarket.

There's never any point in debating with your Pig. It is an animal and must always be treated like one!

HARD TO RECOGNIZE SQUEAL #11

"You know, you've been doing great lately. You've really been taking care of yourself with this 'Cage the Pig' stuff. You're looking and feeling a lot better. Therefore, you're finally thin and healthy enough to get away with a GREAT BIG GIANT HAIRY BINGE!!! Let's just do it, you and me, whaddyasay? Can we? Can we? Huh? PLEEEEEEEEEEASE!!!?" – Your Pig

Let me answer this ridiculous Squeal with a serious question: Is your body a great big garbage can, the sole purpose of which is to process as much refuse as possible? And as soon as enough Pig Slop has been emptied from that canister, are you supposed to rush in and fill it up with more garbage?

—OR—

Or is your body a sacred vessel meant to carry you forward and supply you with energy, peace, and happiness in order to accomplish your goals and live your dreams?

You know the right answer...

And you know the Pig's answer too...

So you know what to do, right? *(Cage the Pig!)*

But if the above is not enough for you to dismiss this ridiculous Pig Squeal then consider a half dozen more analogies:

- If you skipped a month of high school every time you completed one, you'd NEVER graduate...

- If the people who built tall buildings knocked them down every time a few stories were complete then we wouldn't have ANY tall buildings...

- If you stopped peeing every time you squeezed out a few drops your bladder would eventually explode...

- If you decided to get out of bed every night as soon as you got two hours of sleep you'd be psychotically sleep deprived within a few weeks...

- If you built HALF a bridge over a river and encouraged cars to drive over it, they'd plummet to their death...

- And if you let your dog crap on the rug every time he did one good one outside then, well...let's just say I won't be coming to a dinner party at your house any time soon!

There are some projects meant to be taken to completion, and achieving your health and fitness goals should be very high—*if not first!*—on that list.

HARD TO RECOGNIZE SQUEAL #12

"Hold on just a minute now, Bubba! This is about *willpower*, and everyone knows you can't diet on willpower alone. All the latest studies have shown willpower is something you use up as you deal with stress and make decisions throughout the day. See? NOW I've gotcha. I've gotcha....I'VE GOTCHA!!! It's absolutely hopeless to rely on willpower. You're going to Binge. You are. You are. You ARE! And since the time will definitely come, why bother waiting? Let's do it now!!!" – Your Pig

This *is* a tricky Squeal because there's a wealth of evidence which does actually suggest willpower is a limited resource. Deciding between competing alternatives *(like eating junk vs. a healthy meal)* really does tax our mental energy. And so people make increasingly poorer choices as the day goes on and stress wears them down. There are only so many good decisions we can make each day.

On the surface then, it seems willpower may be doomed to fail, and Never Binge Again may be an impossible dream. But when you place these scientific findings *in context* you'll see this idea is just the Pig at work...

The key is understanding willpower is only necessary when there's actually a choice to be made, but when your options are clearly constrained beyond all reasonable doubt, deciding requires virtually no effort at all.

Don't believe me? OK! Time for another thought experiment: How much willpower did it take for you NOT to rob a bank today? Did you spend a lot of the day agonizing about whether or not to do it? Worrying that one day when you're particularly tired and stressed, you just won't have the willpower to resist, even though you didn't rob one today?

Of course not!

Why?

Because you're NOT a bank robber.

You NEVER rob banks, so walking past a bank without robbing it is truly effortless. You have unknowingly made a decision NOT to be a thief as a matter of principle. Thieving is NOT in your character, so it will NEVER take effort for you to resist robbing a bank, regardless of how stressed you may become or how much willpower you may have at any given moment. Why? Because you're a law abiding citizen. You're simply NOT the kind of person who robs banks.

I know the example is a little over the top, so let's bring it down a notch: Do you routinely exert effort to avoid taking the waitress' tips sitting on the counter ad a diner or a restaurant... even when you're sure nobody would see you?

See where I'm going? The point is, you don't have to strain and struggle to resist doing something you've sworn NEVER to do as a matter of character... as long as the line is crystal clear.

Deciding WHAT KIND OF PERSON YOU WANT TO BE OR ARE BECOMING trumps willpower...

Character wins the day.

The situation does become a little more difficult with the CONDITIONALS category of your Food Plan. But only a little, because you can actually translate every conditional into a never.

For example, "I only eat pretzels at baseball games" can become "I NEVER eat pretzels outside of a major league baseball stadium." "I can eat as many calories as I want on the weekends" can be translated to "I NEVER consume more than 2,750 calories per day during the work week."

ALWAYS can be translated to NEVER. For example "I always drink a glass of water as soon as I wake up" becomes "I NEVER leave my bedroom in the morning without drinking a glass of water."

See what I mean?

The trick is making sure every rule in your Food Plan is defined with crystal clarity. If you've got extraordinarily "bright lines" to define the boundaries, then it does NOT take any willpower to recognize and keep to them.

It's only when you've accepted the Pig's desires as actual, viable options that you'll need willpower to resist.

HARD TO HEAR PIG SQUEAL #13
"Just This One Last Time"

Most people are familiar with this Squeal. "Just this one last time", the Pig will say... "We are definitely going to start again tomorrow... so why not? Pleaz???? Can we!!!??"

Like the old proverb says "give an inch and it will take a mile"... that's what your Pig has planned and you know it! Which is why we ALWAYS must use the present moment to be healthy. Every bite counts.

We never give in. Never, ever, ever, ever, ever, EVER!

Always use the present moment to be healthy.

HARD TO HEAR PIG SQUEAL #14
"You Will Be Tortured with Cravings Forever!"

When most people first Cage their Pigs they begin to hear a very loud Squeal to the effect that life will now be nothing more than an unending barrage of misery due to incessant Cravings which are bound to go indefinitely!

But the scientifically proven principle of neuroplasticity rescues us here. What this principle says is that "things that fire together wire together"...

So if you simply withhold the Slop from the Pig for long enough—especially if you substitute something healthier to feed your body's genuine nutritional needs—the brain will neurologically re-wire itself to crave the healthier thing instead.

Take my own experience quitting chocolate, for example. And please note, you don't have to quit chocolate, this is just for illustration.

Anyway, my Pig insisted the chocolate Cravings were going to be intolerable forever. In fact, it threw a whole bunch of ridiculously strong ones at me at first... stronger than I'd ever experienced before. But when I finally understood how Never Binge Again worked and told the Pig I was willing to tolerate ANY level of discomfort without giving in, something kind of miraculous happened...

The Cravings diminished...

First in frequency...

Then in intensity...

Until, about 6 to 8 weeks later, they were almost entirely gone.

It's been several years now that I'm chocolate free *(I don't recall the exact date for reasons covered previously)* and I can't ever remember what it tastes like. I don't WANT to remember either... because it's quite blissful being free... and I know even one bite would re-awaken my Pig on that front.

And my Pig does NOT Squeal about chocolate Cravings in ANY significant way any longer!

The point is, your Pig's notion that you must to keep Binging because the Cravings will otherwise torture you forever is patently false. You're susceptible to this Squeal because you simply haven't abstained long enough for your brain to rewire itself back towards what nature intended...

But now you've got the Never Binge Again method to get through that wall...

And it's a MUCH smaller hurdle than your Pig would have you believe! (As long as you don't reinforce it by eating the Slop... if you do, the clock unfortunately resets.)

HARD TO HEAR PIG SQUEAL #15
"I Can't Get You Now But I Will Definitely Get You Later!"

At some point when I'm working with clients and helping them identify every last Squeal they're tempted to abide by, we get to the point where they feel confident they're not going to Binge right now... but their Pig has them convinced they will definitely Binge LATER. Tomorrow. Next week. At a party. On the Holidays. At someone's birthday party. In a few months when they're too hungry, angry, lonely, or tired. When they become too emotionally upset. Something...

Well, the thing is, your Pig does NOT have a time machine, and the ONLY time you can ever Binge is right now. At all points in the future the will always be NOW. Even as you are reading this and coming to the period in this sentence, the time is once again NOW. And again, now is once again upon us. And NOW too.

The reason this is important is because to Never Binge Again, all you really need to do is Never Binge Now! Since it's ALWAYS now, never binging now translates to never binging forever.

It's a weird line of reasoning but it works to purge the doubt and insecurity generated by the Pig's "I'll get you later" Squeal... and paradoxically that's all it takes to defeat it.

Please note "I Never Binge Now Therefore I Will Never Binge Again" is MUCH different than the "One Day at a Time" philosophy of the 12 step programs. "One Day at a Time" implies "I may binge tomorrow – all I can control is today"... and stems from a philosophy of powerlessness...

Whereas "I Never Binge Now Therefore I Will Never Binge Again" stems from a philosophy of power.

YOU are in control and can confidently declare you will NEVER Binge Again...you are not some pathetic, diseased weakling who can't hope for anything more than one day of abstinence... and who believes relapse must be a part of recovery.

Your Pig does not have a time machine, and all you need to remember is "I Never Binge Now". Period, end of story.

HARD TO HEAR PIG SQUEAL #16
"It's Always Been This Way So It Must Always BE This Way in the Future"

In the past, you may have always given into the Pig eventually. But the past does not determine the future, and if everyone was doomed to do nothing but repeat their past behavior exactly then ALL learning would be impossible. But we know this isn't true. Science, literature, ethics, mathematics... they all consistently progress. As a species we are actually learning machines.

To paraphrase Wayne Dyer, if you've driven 50 miles on Lake Michigan in a motor boat and have a long straight wake that extends behind you in ONE direction only... this says NOTHING about your ability to turn the wheel.

So just turn the wheel and Cage Your Pig!

DETAILED INTERVIEW ON
THE SNEAKY PIG SQUEALS

For a much more detailed discussion of these sneaky Pig Squeals please download the free audio *(and transcript)* "Sneaky Pig Squeals" from www.NeverBingeAgain.com

CHAPTER 12

Discipline vs. Regret

Jim Rohn said "A Life of Discipline is Better Than a Life of Regret," but your Pig vehemently disagrees. It wants you to think discipline restricts your freedom, when precisely the opposite is true.

Most people remember feeling like their whole world opened up when they first got their driver's license. They could finally just get in the car and go anywhere they desired. No longer were they dependent upon others.

But what these very same people forget is that in order to acquire this freedom, they first had to master a series of disciplines. They needed to learn the rules of the road, amass a certain number of supervised driving hours, and pass a written test. Only then could they take the live road test.

The keys to the driving kingdom are *only* given to those who've proven themselves capable of following the rules of the road in earnest. Mastering rules and discipline is how we *increase* freedom in our society, not restrict it!

Here's another way to look at it: Freedom isn't free! It's only for those willing to pay the price.

Your Pig says you're giving up freedom by imposing a disciplined Food Plan, but discipline itself is the price which must be paid for freedom. Without discipline, you will *never* experience the freedom to:

> ➤ Eat without guilt...
>
> ➤ Live in the body of your dreams...
>
> ➤ Live with a minimum of dietary illnesses...
>
> ➤ Have the energy only a truly nourished body can provide...
>
> ➤ Enjoy confidence in your ability to master your own impulses...
>
> ➤ Choose what to eat, when to eat, and where to eat...
>
> ➤ Accomplish progressively more meaningful goals, fully confident you can count on yourself to stay on track until they are achieved...

A disciplined Food Plan doesn't restrict your freedom, it enhances it 100 fold. In actuality it is *the Pig* which seeks to restrict your freedom. If it were given its way you'd be nothing more than a slave to its impulses, and your true freedom would go out the window.

It's your Pig who frames the problem as Freedom _versus_ Discipline in the first place. As if you had to choose one or the other, when in reality freedom ceases to exist in the absence of discipline.

The real question is whether you'll choose a life of discipline versus a life of regret. And when you frame it in this context, it doesn't seem like much of a choice at all, does it?

You know what to do.

(Cage the Pig!)

NO REGRETS WORKSHEET

If you'd like to more clearly see what the Pig may cause you to regret later on, please download the "No Regrets" worksheet. It's part of the free book upgrade available at www.NeverBingeAgain. com

CHAPTER 13

The Psychology of Bingeing, Not Bingeing, and Thinking Too Much About Food

Many years ago when I first started to research food addiction, I wrote a book called "Eat with Your Head™" based in part on a self-funded survey with over 40,000 people on the relationship between personality and Binge food choices.

A few years later my wife and I developed a website called "EmotionalEatingSecrets.com[10]."

At the time, I was very taken with the idea that delving deep into one's personal psychology would yield powerful insight into why any given person Binged. Moreover, I believed it was necessary to acquire such insights in order to stop.

But now, many years later, I know I was unequivocally wrong!

---

[10] While I promptly removed the "Eat with Your Head" book from the market once I realized how wrongheaded my original notions about psychology and food addiction were, I was unable to do the same with the EmotionalEatingSecrets.com website because it is intricately bound up with other projects and partners to whom I have legal commitments.

It may be intriguing and psychologically valuable to figure out why your Pig prefers chocolate and pizza while other people's Pigs like donuts and potato chips, why you chose to let your Pig have its Slop in private while others prefer to Binge in the company of others, why anger triggers some people to Binge and loneliness triggers others, etc...

But the notion it's necessary to answer these kinds of questions before you can stop Bingeing is 100% Pig Squeal. From the Pig's perspective:

> "You know, Mama and Papa didn't love us nearly enough. They said and did some pretty awful things. And everyone deserves love, right? Oh well. I guess we'll just have to keep Bingeing to fill that big empty hole Mama and Papa left deep inside us. At least until ALL the tragic events from our past have been uncovered and we can find healthy substitutes for the love we missed out on. I know, I know, Pig Slop can't ever replace Mommy and Daddy's love. But it sure does taste good. Too bad, so sad. Let's Binge!!!" – Your Pig

Or alternatively:

> "Our life is just too stressful. And our loved ones don't support our personal goals and dreams nearly enough. All we have to rely on in this world is Pig Slop. Maybe we'll be able to stop eating it when we have less stress or better coping mechanisms. But for now, we simply MUST Binge in order to cope. Ooooooooooh!!! Ooooooooooh!!! Ooooooooooh!!! How yummy!!!!" – Your Pig

Now, please don't get me wrong, I thoroughly support psychological and spiritual soul searching. In fact, a big part of the reason I myself have such a meaningful life is because of the years I've spent with therapists, coaches, and mentors digging deep into my own thoughts, feelings, and past experiences. I wouldn't give it up for the world.

But soul searching has absolutely nothing to do with your ability to quit Bingeing. Zero. Nada. Zilch.

This is a ridiculously simple concept which shouldn't have to be written—but because of the confusing culture in which we live I'm afraid it does...

You do NOT need to know why you Binge. You just need to stop.

It doesn't matter whether it's because nobody came to your fourth grade bowling party, because you saw your Momma in her underwear, or because grandpa forgot to pick you up at school when you were five.

You know how to eat healthy.

You know how to construct an unambiguous Food Plan, making well-considered, intellectual decisions to balance the tradeoff between short vs. long term gratification and health.

You know what a Binge is and what a Binge isn't.

So just don't Binge again...

Ever.

Even if everyone you love suddenly dies.

Even if you feel justifiably lonely, alienated, angry, depressed, anxious, and/or stressed beyond all hope and reason...

Just *Never Binge Again!*

Now, if you want to do some soul searching to see why you were convincible to start Bingeing at a particular time and circumstance in your life...

Fine. More power to you.

But you don't need to wait for a good answer before you stop Bingeing.

You don't need to see a Shrink to stop Bingeing.

To stop, just draw 100% clear lines and stop.

That's ALL you need to know about the psychology of Bingeing.

It really *is* that simple.

While Binges are often associated with emotional experiences—*and therefore serve as an excellent jumping off point for soulful exploration*—they do NOT and cannot CAUSE you to Binge!

The notion that emotional upset *causes* Binges is actually harmful, because it gives the Pig license to keep Bingeing until the upset is over and/or fully understood.

Remember, this is coming from a guy with a Ph.D. in psychology—*who grew up in a family of psychologists and therapists and still thinks of himself as a psychologist first and foremost*—so I don't say this lightly!

Bingeing transforms you into a wild animal. It rejects the laws of humanity and returns you to the jungle where life is brutish, chaotic, and short.

Bingeing wipes out your spirit.

Don't spend years investigating WHY you Binge before you stop. Just stop.

Choose to stand for the domination of the human spirit over our animal nature so you can accomplish your dreams and pass your experiences on to your loved ones.

Which leads me to one last point about the psychology of Bingeing...

It's NOT a foregone conclusion that childhood adversity will traumatize a person and set them on a path of compulsive self-destruction. In fact, adversity *can* result in both a strength of character AND a determined persistence to right the wrongs one has experienced.

Yes, there are victims of child abuse who wind up abusing drugs or becoming serious binge eaters. And there are those who choose to perpetuate the abuse cycle by victimizing their own children...

But there are also those who turn into incredibly gentle souls, passionate about helping others who've been through anything similar.

We all must make a decision in this life to either get well or get even.

Bingeing is glued to the revenge journey...

Your resolve to Never Binge Again puts you on the royal road to forgiveness and wellbeing.

To partake of everything life has to offer...

Cage the Pig!

ONE MORE THING AND IT'S IMPORTANT...

Even though you do NOT need to know why you Binge to stop, and even though you CAN do it on your own... the practical implementation of the Never Binge Again method often goes more quickly *(and is more successful)* with assistance from those trained and/or experienced in the method...

For this reason I DO offer a coaching program at a very affordable rate *(www.NeverBingeAgainCoaching.com)*. We can help you customize your Food Plan to work for you in particular, no matter how much you travel, eat out, no matter how much stress you experience, how many children and/or uncooperative spouses you may have... even at night, on weekends, or when your emotions are utterly out of control. www.NeverBingeAgainCoaching.com

CHAPTER 14

A Radical View
on Guilt and Shame

We've talked about this throughout the book in order to quiet your Pig enough so you could actually read it. In this short chapter, I want to put to rest any remaining fear you may have of guilt or shame for having made a mistake.

I've run into many people who say the Never Binge Again approach very much appeals to them, but they won't implement it because they fear a "guilt hangover" when they inevitably find themselves Bingeing again. But if you've been paying attention, you should recognize this as just another Pig Squeal:

> "Don't bother committing to a Food Plan because you can't ever hope to do it perfectly, and then I'll beat you up and make you feel horribly guilty...so you never try such a silly thing again. C'mon, are you really going to do this nonsense? Let's just Binge!!!" – Sincerely, Your Pig

See, the Pig has a plan for you to *FAIL*.

But YOU have a plan to *SUCCEED*.

Just remember this distinction and ignore that vile creature.

The natural, healthy purpose of guilt and shame is to draw your attention to a bad behavior so you can correct it. Therefore, once you've made a 100% firm plan to never Binge again, there's absolutely NO purpose to holding onto your guilt or shame.

Guilt and shame about Bingeing are uncomfortable emotions which quickly dissipate in the absence of a plan to Binge again. Much like the pain you feel after touching a hot stove, these feelings exist to help you learn...and they go away quickly once you've done so.

You don't need to walk around for a month beating yourself up for touching the stove, you just say "I'll Never Do That Again"... and once you're 100% convinced of your commitment, you easily let it go.

Unfortunately the field of psychology has gone too far in its attempt to eliminate the guilt and shame which Victorian times imposed upon us for our natural human feelings *(mostly sexuality and anger)*...

And today popular wisdom suggests we should eradicate these emotions entirely...

But that's NOT entirely healthy either.

We should actually WANT to feel guilty when we break our commitments... or else we'd be removing our motivation to change, and denigrating the meaning of our word.

But we must also be willing to let go of these uncomfortable emotions once we've analyzed what went wrong and made a commitment to correct it in the future...

Holding onto guilt and shame for a well-analyzed and corrected mistake is the Pig's way of doing penance in advance for its plan to Binge again.

Don't let your Pig talk you into fearing your guilt...

Or hold onto it once you've fixed the problem.

Touching a hot stove is painful...

And food mistakes do burn indeed ...

But if you're a human being who's still breathing, you've got a miraculously strong ability to recover and leave that mistake in the past.

Cage the Pig and watch how fast it loses power!

CHAPTER 15

"Unconscious" Bingeing

The Pig always prefers us to remain 100% unaware of its activities because it knows that if we were fully aware of what it was up to, we would have to be crazy to give it ANY control! For this reason, most people report feeling somewhat "unconscious" during a Binge, almost as if another entity had "taken over." Some people even suggest this went on for weeks or even months, and they simply "woke up" having gained a lot of weight and feeling miserable...

But it's more accurate and helpful to say we consciously decided not to think about what we were doing during a Binge. We turned a blind eye so the Pig could have its Slop. We did NOT go into a temporary coma while the Pig did its thing!

Here's what I mean...

If I were to interview you immediately after a Binge, the odds are very good you'd be able to recount virtually everything which happened. We could reconstruct exactly what you ate, what brands you bought, what the bags and boxes looked like, about how much you paid for them, where you got them, what the cashier looked like, what else was in the isles where you picked up the junk, how you decided what to buy, about how much you put in your cart *(or arms)*... and if we tried hard enough you could even remember the stream of thoughts which led you to the store.

The video recorder in your mind was running the whole time you were bingeing... you just chose not to look through the lens while it was making the tape.

While it's only natural to behave like this because it's too uncomfortable for a rational, conscious person to accept they are allowing themselves to be out of control, it's still a critically important distinction.

The notion of being unconscious may provide a safe haven from the guilt and shame we feel about the Binge, but it does so at a very steep price...

To believe the Pig has the ability to knock you unconscious so it can do as it pleases is to relinquish your free will and responsibility. To believe the Pig can put you in a coma removes all your power and ability to keep your own word...

And it's your word that allows you to set and achieve goals...

To accomplish the things you want to in this life...

To be true to the people you love...

To be exactly the kind of person you want to be.

Remember, you can and should let go of the guilt and shame associated with Bingeing once you've analyzed the Squeals, corrected your Food Plan *(if necessary,)* and re-committed 100%...

So you really don't need the cover of a weird "psychological anesthesia" for your past Binge behaviors. You are never going to binge again, so you can and should claim responsibility for every last choice you made in the past.

This way the Pig will know you're always watching...

And are prepared to dominate it if it even *thinks* about getting out of line.

CHAPTER 16

Your New Best Friend

I'd like to introduce you to your new best friend, the bathroom scale.

> "The *$@%##!! scale - are you *$@%##!! Kidding me!?? Are you really going to let that thing rule our lives? C'mon... we don't need no *$@%##!! scale! We can tell what we weigh from how we look in the mirror and how our clothes feel. Besides, it's NO fun eating Pig Slop when we have to weigh in the next day, right? Ooooooooooh – Pig Slop – let's go get us some Pig Slop! Can we? Can we? Pleeeeeeeeeeeeeeeeeeeeeeeease!!!!???"

In this life, information is power. It's better to know than not to know.

Stephen Covey points out a commercial airplane is actually *off course* 99% of the time it flies from New York to Los Angeles! Despite this, the craft reaches its destination every time. How? The pilots consistently monitor their instruments and make small adjustments throughout the flight.

So what do pilots know which our Pigs desperately fear?

It's a LOT easier to make dozens, or even hundreds of tiny course corrections all along your journey than to ignore the feedback and find yourself thousands of miles from where you'd hoped to land later on!

Think of your scale as one of those critical "airplane instruments." Faithfully take the feedback it provides you with each morning. Interpret the data objectively, and adjust your food and exercise accordingly. It's that simple.

But, see, your Pig has other plans:

How Your Pig Tries to Keep You Away from a Daily Weigh In

Pig Squeal	Healthy Thought
There are too many factors which influence what you weigh each morning. How much salt did you have yesterday? How late did you eat at night? Did you exercise? When? Did you have a morning B.M. or not? Was it BIG enough? Did you get all the pee out? What did you have for dinner? Do you have your period? Maybe we should go spend a little more time trying to "fully empty ourselves out" first. Wait – we don't have time for that. *(We definitely DO have time for Pig Slop though... Yummy!!!)*	Ask any statistician—they'll confirm that in order to determine how each of these factors genuinely influences your weight you'll require *hundreds* of weigh-ins. By preventing you from *consistently* stepping onto the scale, your Pig removes your power to see real trends in loss or gain over time. See, any given weigh-in means very little. It's the trend that counts. How your average weight changes as the months go by...and there's NO way to know that if you don't weigh in regularly.
If you rush home after a binge and weigh yourself to find you've only gained one pound, well, that'll just encourage you to binge more. You need to let the consequences of our Binges mount so maybe someday you'll finally see the light. Of course, until then, we can Binge right!!!?	Your Pig wants to be sure you don't catch and stop the small gains. It wants to keep you in the dark until the weight gain is absolutely impossible to ignore so it can maximize its Binge time. Poor Pig. Weigh yourself regularly and Cage the Pig!

The scale is just a number. Are you really going to let it define us? Do we really want to look at it every day and feel bad about ourselves?	Your mortgage statement is just a number too...but if you ignore it I'm pretty sure the bank will eventually take your house away. The speed limit is just a number too, but if you ignore it you can get into a lot of trouble. The thing of it is, these numbers *exist* whether you look at them or not. By NOT looking you're letting the scale define you. By looking *you* take control and put the scale in its rightful place.
What about body fat!!! You've been lifting weights, doing a lot of working out, etc... and that isn't reflected on the scale. The scale could be higher because you've gained a lot of muscle!	It's extremely difficult to put on more than one pound of muscle per month. Over the course of a year you MIGHT be able to add 15 pounds of genuine muscle. But if you have a bunch of fat to lose and you genuinely are losing it, the odds are your fat loss will outpace your muscle gain by a factor of at least 4 to 1. Most body builders will also tell you it's also very difficult to both lose weight and gain muscle at the same time. Bottom line? If your Food Plan is effective at burning fat for you AND you weigh yourself consistently, the scale should be trending down week by week *(or at least month by month)*. If it's not, no biggie... it just means it's time for an adjustment.

You can't spend all day obsessing about what the scale says. You've got to live your life, don't you?	You can't spend all your time driving with your eyes on the speedometer either... it's just one of the many things you scan as you go about navigating the road. But we're NOT going to put a piece of cardboard over the speedometer and pretend it doesn't exist while you drive, are we? The scale is just one more data point you effortlessly scan each morning to help you navigate your day... not something to obsess about, and not something to ignore.
If the scale has GOOD news you can just use it as a rationale to Binge	Your Pig WANTS you to Binge when the scale gets low enough because it sees your health as a great big garbage can to fill with Pig Slop the moment there's room. But YOU see your body as a sacred vessel and the most amazing thing you'll ever own. There are MANY ways to celebrate good news...*Binging is NOT one of them!*
If we haven't weighed ourselves in a while and the scale has BAD news... I'll just point out how pathetic you are and ask when you're going to finally just give up and be "a happy fat person." So you absolutely can't weigh yourself if you don't want that to happen. Oh, and by the way, since we have no idea what we weigh then there's no harm in having a little Pig Slop now and then, is there?	Not weighing yourself for long periods of time is kind of like driving a car with your eyes closed. Even if you know the neighborhood really well, the odds are pretty good you're not going to get *too* far without crashing! And having worked with many overweight clients I can tell you the idea of a "happy fat person" is mostly an illusion. (*Despite our culture's warped notions about what constitutes beauty, there are too just many health, energy, relationship, and other issues associated with excess weight which take their toll on the individual's sense of freedom, power, and the ability to enjoy life.*)

Most of the permanently thin people I've ever known have told me the best way they ever found to lose weight was a regular weigh-in. Why? Because this made it next to impossible for their Pigs to keep fooling them about the impact of their Pig Slop.

In my experience, most people do best to weigh-in first thing in the morning, because it forces a reality check BEFORE you start your daily food intake.

Make friends with your scale. Give it a great big hug and a kiss each morning to thank it for its consistent, simple willingness to tell you what's going on. Try saying this now "I love you scale. I really, really love you. You are my best friend forever."

No?

OK, then just get on the damn scale each morning without fail, no matter what your Pig's emotional reaction may be. I'll bet you'll like what happens in the long run, and it will make your Pig truly miserable.

Poor Pig.

Cage the Pig!

PS – Some people prefer a less-frequent-but-still-regular weigh in. Maybe once a week or once a month. Just like everything else in the Never Binge Again way of life this is, in fact, 100% completely and totally up to YOU. But in my experience, less regular weigh-ins allow more room for Pig Parties in between. Just sayin'

PPS – Many people find it helpful to make their own written list of EVERYTHING their Pig may say to sabotage them in EVERY weigh in scenario. This includes things your Pig likes to Squeal about when the number is too high, too low, and just right. *(Your Pig will seize EVERY opportunity to convince you to Binge – writing out these scenarios ahead of time will ensure you recognize the Squeals)*

CHAPTER 17

YourPersonal Pig Squeal Journal

As discussed above, all that's necessary to stop Bingeing is to stop Bingeing...

Define a Food Plan, commit to it with a 100% certain resolution, and then go about the rest of your life.

You don't have to practice using any particular tools, meditations, chants, or rituals. All you need to do is comply with your Food Plan, and utterly ignore any thought *(Pig Squeal)* which suggests you do otherwise.

Journaling is therefore NOT a requirement of the Never Binge Again program.

That said, you can only ignore Pig Squeal if you recognize it. And— *especially in the beginning*—the Pig will be busy dreaming up NEW ways to disguise its Squeals. After all, the Pig doesn't want to be locked in a cage forever. It will passionately work to find loopholes.

Ultimately all the Pig's reasons boil down to "because it tastes good" or "because I want the Food High"...and it will eventually stop bothering you when it realizes you know this. Like all wild animals in captivity it realizes there's no use continuing to bang on the inside of a permanently locked door.

But because the Pig lives inside you and has access to your native thinking, every person will hear different types of Pig Squeal during the adjustment phase...so it's impossible to list every last possibility in this book.

For this reason journaling can be very helpful.

Journaling sensitizes you to how the Pig sounds when it attempts a new Squeal. Wait, what's that? I can hear your Pig now:

> "Glenn says you've got to journal or else you won't hear my super-creative NEW reasons for Bingeing. This means the first day you forget and/or don't have the time to journal we can go off to the races and Binge our little faces off. Yippeee!!!"

Pig Squeal!

You've unambiguously defined a Food Plan which draws clear lines in the sand...

You've solemnly sworn an oath to hold to it forever...

You CAN do this regardless of whether you journal or not.

But journaling makes it less stressful because you'll recognize the Squeals sooner. That's all.

Anyway, a simple way to go about this is to challenge your Pig each morning before you've eaten anything. Say "Go ahead Pig. I'll give you control over my fingers to type/write any reason you can think of to convince me to feed you some Slop. Let's see if you can come up with a good one!"

It's OK. They're your fingers and you can take back control whenever you like. And because you will NEVER Binge again no matter what the Pig says, you can let the Pig have at it.

Once the Pig's Squeals are in black and white it takes less energy to recognize and ignore them.

Now, you'd think the Pig would catch on to this game and just stop playing after it realizes you're only baiting it to reveal its hand. But the Pig is so impulse driven it can't help but lunge at the opportunity. Again and again, no matter what the results were last time, the time before that, or the forty two million times before *that!*

It's kind of like dangling roast beef in front of a Doberman Pincher. The chance to get the meat, however slim, is too alluring. Its primitive instincts will take over, no matter what happened before.

Just like the Doberman, your Pig will always give you its best shot if you dangle a Bingeing opportunity in front of it.

Stupid Pig.

Cage it!

CHAPTER 18

Binge Anxiety

Many people say they feel frightened a Binge is imminent and/or inevitable "someday soon" shortly after resolving to Never Binge Again. These people aren't consciously lying, they just don't realize it's the Pig talking, not them.

What's underneath "I'm afraid I might Binge" is just the Pig saying "I really, really want to Binge!"

Always.

100% of the time.

It's that simple.

Binge Anxiety is a big hairy lie which starts and ends with the Pig's plan to Binge...

Any and all doubt in your ability to Never Binge Again is Pig Squeal.

Any and all insecurity comes from the Pig.

But you will Never Binge Again, so you can just put this to rest.

WHAT TO DO WITH BINGE ANXIETY?

I've prepared a simple Binge Anxiety audio and wallet-cheat-card you can download and carry around with you in your smart phone. Get it at www.NeverBingeAgain.com

CHAPTER 19

What to Do
When It's Not Working

"What if it doesn't work?"

This question *itself* is Pig Squeal.

By definition, the Never Binge Again approach isolates and starves any and all Binge-related impulses so you can once again exercise free will with food. How you use that innate human capacity is entirely up to you.

If you choose to deploy free will to work for you, it WILL work for you. You literally can't fail, because all you're doing is letting go of an illusion and stepping squarely into the way things are.

If you choose to consciously and purposefully let the Pig out of its cage now that you know it's game, well, that's up to you too...

See, Never Binge Again is about restoring your sense of free will and power. It's a fiercely independent philosophy...

You definitely CAN cage the Pig forever – but you're the ONLY one who can.

If it works for you, I won't take credit...

But if it doesn't work, I won't take the blame either...

Because all I've really done is point out that YOU were in control all along.

I gave you permission to make your own Food Plan—*(as if you really needed that from me?)*—and a way to more clearly hear your Pig Squealing...

But the truth is, you were in Kansas all along, Dorothy!

All you needed to do was click your heals, open your eyes, and sharpen your thinking about Pig Slop. You needed to stop listening to the insanity about food in our culture, to take a hard look at what the food industry was doing to you, and to decide for yourself what belongs in vs. out of your own body.

I really do hope I've opened your eyes and empowered you...

And most importantly, I hope you now realize your Pig is NOT You!!!

But if you're repeatedly struggling there are a few extra steps you might want to take...

First, consider a Food Plan which doesn't include any refined sugar, flour, or alcohol. None. Because these substances destabilize the body in a multitude of ways which create progressively more cravings for themselves.

Now, I'm NOT by any stretch of the imagination saying everyone must eliminate them...

But it's the rare doctor indeed who'll tell you "the reason you're not healthy is because you need more refined sugar, flour, and alcohol", know what I mean?

Never is a lot easier than sometimes for a LOT of people with these modern drugs.

OK, enough said.

Before we leave this chapter I'd like to mention one last ploy your Pig may use in a last-ditch attempt to trick you, and I want to explain it to you before we wind down our time together in this crazy little book I wrote...

And here it is:

> "You can't stop Bingeing using free will because free will doesn't exist." – *Your Pig's last ditch attempt*

What's going on here in your Pig's last ditch attempt to get you to dislodge your jaw and empty a delicatessen into it is a bit subtle...

See, the Pig wants to draw you into an unresolvable debate so you'll keep Bingeing until a definitive answer is found.

Now, although I'm not intellectually equipped with decades of philosophical study to prove it, I emphatically DO believe free will exists. But even if it didn't and our fate was entirely predetermined, what evidence would we have to conclude we were fated to exercise the Pig's desires vs. our own?

See, the Pig is hiding the second half of its argument in the anti-free-will ploy. What it's really saying is because there's no free will you must *choose* to let it keep Bingeing. But if there were no free will, you couldn't choose anything at all.

I mean, maybe God wound up the universe and pre-determined we would all eat nothing but lettuce for the entirety of our lives. We really have NO way of knowing... despite what our Pigs may say. *(Note: In the end, I'm one of the most agnostic people you'll ever meet so please take this for what it's worth...but there's an interesting passage in Genesis 1:29 for anyone who's interested in what the Bible has to say about what we're supposed to eat)*

In any case, the answer to this particularly tricky Squeal is to let the philosophers debate the free will issue until they're blue in the face...

Because even if free will didn't exist we'd still have to act as if it did or we couldn't have a society at all—*because nobody would be responsible for anything, and anyone could do whatever they wanted without justifiable consequence or punishment!*

Until someone has had a scientifically demonstrable and repeatable talk with God *(whatever that means)* we will probably never know. In the meantime, we'll just relentlessly continue to dominate the Pig...

Why?

Because we can.

CHAPTER 20

Alcohol Pigs, Drug Pigs, and Other Pigs Worth Dominating

B y now, if you've implemented even just a little of what we've talked about I'm sure your brain is exploding with ideas for applying the Never Binge Again philosophy to other areas of your life.

The truth is, I didn't invent the idea of aggressively separating your thin-thinking-self from your fat-thinking-alter-ego, then carefully watching for the latter so you could ignore it with contempt. The "devil vs. angel on your shoulder" has been man's way of wrestling with constructive vs. destructive impulses since time immemorial.

But while others have been hard at work for decades perfecting its application to black-and-white addictions like drugs, alcohol, and cigarettes, I found serious modifications were necessary to apply this thinking to complex behavioral systems like overeating.

Most significantly it was necessary to develop a more appropriate before-vs. after-the-Binge mindset. This was necessary to address the multitude of attempts most people seem to require in order to *"confidently pedal to the top the Never Binge Again hill"* without becoming distracted by the possibility of failure and/or the destructive use of guilt and shame for mistakes.

It was also critical to identify an appropriate analogy—*society's reliance on a body of law*—for complex behavioral systems as compared to simple yes/no addictions.

And finally, it was necessary to develop a set of core principles for defining an individual's Food Plan without usurping their autonomy.

Now, if you DO struggle with drugs, alcohol, or other black-and-white addictions, I can't recommend anyone's work more highly than Jack Trimpey's at Rational Recovery Systems. (*www.Rational.org*) Rather than trying to define an "Alcohol Pig" or "Drug Pig", please just use his methodology, which you'll find very compatible with the philosophy you've learned in this book.

While there is some overlap, these black and white addictions will NOT succumb to the Never Binge Again philosophy I've outlined in this book in the same way that food will. I've also never seriously struggled with drugs, alcohol, or cigarettes on a personal level. More importantly, I haven't studied those addictions in the same comprehensive way I've studied food.

For these reasons, you're MUCH better off with Mr. Trimpey's body of work if these particular substances have you caught in the Venus Fly Trap of toxic pleasure.

On the other hand, if you're thinking Never Binge Again can be effectively applied to *other* complex behavioral systems in the same way it works for overeating—you're right!

For example, perhaps you'd like to Never Procrastinate Again™ so you can comply 100% with your exercise routine, finish your book, and/or do anything else you know you'd be capable of if it weren't for the self-sabotaging voice inside you which always says "later." Just define a reasonable schedule with 100% clarity, then summarily ignore your Procrastination Pig when it suggests you deviate for any reason whatsoever.

Better yet, read my next book "The End of Failure™" so you can assure yourself of success across every important area of your life going forward and...Never Fail Again. I'm just saying! *(When you download the free bonus materials for Never Binge Again you'll also be sure to be notified when the new book is released. www. NeverBingeAgain.com)*

CHAPTER 21

My Personal Food Plan

What do I eat? None of your Pig's business!

But I will tell you what I will NEVER eat again...

Pig Slop!

CHAPTER 22

The Practical
Course Most People Take

If you've read this far, you know it's entirely possible to make a Food Plan, stick to it, and Never Binge Again. The clarify, focus, and structure this weird trick of mind provides you is enough to purge your mind of the energy-and-confidence-draining power of doubt and insecurity so you can control your eating like never before.

Still—and you should definitely cover your Pig's ears and eyes for this next part—most people DO make mistakes as they are experimenting with the method...

And your Pig will say this proves the method itself is invalid...

That you'll just have to "find something else."

Which is why I talk to a lot of people who say they've TRIED Never Binge Again with SOME success... but they really don't think it can "Work" for them in the long run...and they want to try "something else."

I'm always a little puzzled by this very strange idea. You see, Never Binge Again is NOT like a gastric bypass, a pharmaceutical pill, or a therapeutic "treatment." It's NOT something I do TO you or FOR you to MAKE you stop Bingeing...it's just the systematic application of common sense, free will, and responsibility in a ruthless manner:

First we systematically and ruthlessly identify all your trigger foods and eating behaviors...

Then we clarify the healthiest decisions you can possibly make when confronted by them...

We commit to those decisions as a matter of character *(the kind of person you are or the kind of person you are becoming)*

And we define ANY thought or feeling which suggests we will ever act in the most remote way otherwise as our destructive self *(Pig, Junkyard Dog, etc)*...

This simple set of common sense techniques then clarifies our thinking enough that we can purge our minds of doubt and uncertainty so we can concentrate 100% of our effort on the goal.

If we happen to make a mistake we just get up and refocus our minds once again with 100% effort, just like an Olympic Archer re-focuses on the bulls-eye with crystal clear vision at every pull of the arrow...

And if you DO keep getting up, your aim MUST improve!

The ONLY way to fail at Never Binge Again is to either reject common sense or consciously choose to let the Pig out of its Cage...

And so I always ask people who say "It's not working"...

WHAT IS THE ALTERNATIVE?

Would it be better to shoot for a fuzzy goal? To play "blind archery" and NOT define what healthy eating is for yourself? I don't think so! My grandfather always said "if you don't know where you're going you'll probably wind up someplace else!"

Should we avoid clarifying what a healthy food thought is vs. a destructive one? I can't see how that does anyone any good... you've got to recognize the healthy ones to act on them and the unhealthy ones to avoid them, right?

Should we just "try to eat healthy" and do the best we can? Well, if that worked for you I don't think you'd be reading this!

Should we seek out some new diet guru for the forty seven millionth time? Well, read their books if you want to... but in the end you STILL have to embrace their very specific set of Food Rules and learn how to catch yourself trying to talk yourself out of following it, don't you?

Should we disclaim all responsibility and power over our ability to control ourselves and pretend we have some mysterious, chronic, progressive disease... then spend our lives confessing our troubles in the town square with other helpless people who have this fake disease too? Should we spend nights away from our families talking about how we just can't control ourselves and need to cultivate fear of our own healthy appetites? That would be a VERY dismal view of humanity, don't you think? To say "we can't control ourselves with food" is really to say we are nothing more than animals...and I think human beings are MUCH more than that, don't you?

I SAY NO THANK YOU!!!!

But I understand why people are afraid to be disappointed.

I feel their pain because I previously tried a thousand times and failed.

But if you adopt the attitude of playing the 'never binge again' game...and resolve to be 100% committed to your food plan and caging the pig but are forgiving to yourself and resume the 'never binge again' game if you make a mistake...

Then there is literally NO way to 'fail'... you can only STUMBLE...and if you keep getting up the 'never binge again' way of life virtually

MUST take over your thinking completely so you can truly think like a permanently thin person.

Think of it this way...

There was a time in your life when you didn't know how to walk. You got up, took a few steps and fell right down again. Sometimes right on your face!

Did you give up then and say "this walking thing obviously doesn't work so we'll have to find some other way to get around?"

Of course not.

So enough with the Pig's B.S. already and let's just get on with it!

Your Pig may win a battle or two in the beginning...but it will NOT win the war unless you consciously choose to let it.

Am I right or am I right?

You may not be perfect, but that doesn't mean you can't AIM for perfection. In fact, that's the ONLY way, in my experience, to put the Pig in its Cage for good.

CHAPTER 23

Taking the Next Step

You have everything you need to Never Binge Again right here in this book. You don't have to talk to a shrink, attend a recovery group, smack yourself in the head with a spatula to atone for your mistakes, or go sit by the river for months to contemplate your navel.

You only need to define a healthy Food Plan, commit to it 100%, and remember that Pig Slop is anything even 0.0000001% outside your plan.

Then just ignore the Pig when it Squeals for Slop. Every last time!

Do this and your last Binge—*whether it was 5 seconds, 5 minutes, or 5 months ago*—really can be your LAST.

Notwithstanding the above, some people find it helpful to talk this over in person, absorb the information in a more customized manner in a LIVE environment, and/or see how I help other people with their own Pigs. And some people simply do better when they absorb information in a multitude of formats.

I therefore offer:

> **Never Binge Again Coaching:** Personal help to customize your Food Plan, Ignore the Pig Squeals, and Cage Your Pig for good! www.NeverBingeAgainCoaching.com

> **Personal Consultations**: Get powerful, personalized guidance to stop bingeing right away. Available from myself personally on a very limited basis. Inquire with support via the contact form on www.NeverBingeAgain.com

> **Weekend Immersions**: Make Never Bingeing Again your first priority this month by attending one of our Intensive Food Plan Confidence weekends.

Please visit www.NeverBingeAgain.com **for the latest options. And be sure to download the special FREE book upgrade which contains ALL of the following:**

> **Pig Damage Calculator:** Take the short, free test and see how much impact has the Pig has had on your life. A great way to get motivated and get started.

> **Free Starter Food Plan Templates**: No matter what your nutritional philosophy you'll find a pre-filled starter template to help fill in your own Food Plan with NEVERS, ALWAYS, UNCONDITIONALS, and CONDITIONALS

> **Custom Food Plan Creation Worksheet**: A set of detailed questions to help you identify and customize your own plan.

> **Craving Defeater Set:** Quickly defeat ANY craving with this simple cheat-card you can carry around in your wallet AND and MP3 audio you can play on your smart phone

> **Binge Recovery Set**: This MP3 and Workbook will help you put the Pig back in its cage for good no matter how painful a Binge you've experienced

- **How to Change Your Food Plan Cheat Sheet**: A simple one-pager with a detailed set of criteria to help ensure it's YOU and not your Pig suggesting the changes!

- **Avoiding the Deprivation Trap Workbook:** Struggling with whether to set a particular Food Rule or move a conditional to a NEVER? Who will be deprived, you or your Pig? Fill out this workbook and find out so you can make the decision more easily.

- **The Four Most Common Food Industry Lies and How to Defeat Them *(Audio Interview + Transcript):*** Our society is set up to feed your Pig. Here are some tricky ways they do it, and simple strategies for winning the game regardless!

- **Unusual Ways to Neutralize Other People's Pigs *(Audio Interview + Transcript):*** Troubled by what other people say, do, or tempt you with in an eating environment? Stop that! Just listen to this educational audio and arm yourself with a simple way to immediately neutralize their power

- **12 Sneaky Pig Squeals and How to Defeat Them *(Audio Interview + Transcript):*** Taken directly from people's sneakiest Pigs, this interview will strengthen your ability to recognize Pig Squeal in all its sneaky forms

- **The "No Regrets" Worksheet:** How to see the road not taken – the two different paths and where they may lead

- **Binge Anxiety Killer:** I've prepared a simple Binge Anxiety audio and wallet-sized-cheat-card you can download and carry around with you in your smart phone to help eliminate Binge Anxiety whenever it strikes.

Download All of the Above
in the FREE Book Upgrade at
www.NeverBingeAgain.com

Personal Coaching
www.NeverBingeAgainCoaching.com

Reader's Forum
www.NeverBingeAgainForum.com

Last, I LOVE to hear your stories. It's particularly helpful if you can share sneaky Pig Squeals you've learned to identify. Please post them on our Facebook Page and/or upload them to YouTube and send us the link. Instructions are on the website.

Now, YOU...

Cage the Pig, keep it there and...

Never Binge Again!

Made in the USA
San Bernardino, CA
24 August 2018